Health Is Number One™

Maximizing Your Health

By Craig M. Wax, DO
"America's Family Physician"

Alethos Press, St. Paul, MN

Alethos Press, St Paul, MN

Health Is Number One: Maximizing Your Health

Print ISBN: 979-8-9863314-9-2
eBook ISBN: 979-8-9999301-0-1

Disclaimer:

This book is intended for general information purposes only, not to engender a patient-physician relationship. The health information presented here is for your consideration and edification, not to be considered medical advice. Please consult your trusted independent family physician with any questions and to help you in your best healthy life journey.

–Craig M. Wax, DO

Cover Design by: Craig M. Wax, DO and Alethos Press

Printed in the U.S.A. by Bethany Press International, Bloomington, MN

https://HealthIsNumberOne.com

10 9 8 7 6 5 4 3 2

Table of Contents

Health Is Number One: Maximizing Your Health

Dedication

This work is dedicated to all those who believed in me and the concepts that I have assembled here, my wife, kids, friends, and patients. Further, it is dedicated to the memory of my parents and grandparents who endured and persevered to raise up the next generation. I must acknowledge Paul J. Stankard, studio glass craft artist and friend, for riding me to finally finish the book.

Furthermore, it is dedicated to Andrew Taylor Still, D.O., Robert Thorpe, D.O., and all my mentors, for they showed me the forest and the trees and the intrinsic wisdom of the human body.

–Craig M. Wax, DO

"A student of life must take in each part of the body and study its uses and relations to other parts and systems."

"Nature has supplied her own forces, and man has only to find and apply them."

– Andrew Taylor Still, DO

Editor's Confession

Dr. Craig Wax called to ask if I might be able to help him with this book. He explained that he had worked on it "on and off" for 25 years. Although Dr. Wax had written and published many articles and editorials during that time, the book lay unfinished. After some back-and-forth, we agreed to move ahead together.

In the past, I've helped several brilliant people "fix" their book and then take it through to publication. Most of these authors had good messages that needed to be heard. I had accumulated enough knowledge to provide "additive" material, that is, material to improve the content and usefulness of their message.

Otherwise, working on those books became a work project. (When I help an author from "word one"–that is, I write the book for the author–my interest piques.)

Then I started working on this book. Every chapter spoke to me, so much so that I'd have to share what I learned with my wife of 58 years each time I saw her after leaving my office. She begged me to stop learning because it meant we'd have to change a lifetime of unhealthy behaviors. Perish the thought.

In self-defense, there are at least two or three principles taught in this book that I had already incorporated into my daily practice. All the others, however, and it is a long list, forced me to rethink my lifestyle.

When a book (in my case, a work project) gets to your core, you know it is a necessary book. I am grateful to Dr. Wax for writing it, and thankful to reap the benefits from it.

Be forewarned. You're not going to readily accept Dr. Wax's diagnosis (Dx), his treatment (Tx), or his prescription for health (Rx). With an open mind and a desire to overcome your ailments, and a goal of a longer, healthier life, I believe you will be glad you read it.

Oh, by the way, this is a book that requires a highlighter, a pen, or a pencil to take marginal notes, and perhaps a journal to keep track of your progress.

–Dave Racer, MLitt (2025)
Publisher and Editor
Alethos Press, St. Paul, MN
https://daveracer.com

Foreword

Do you have a loved one who is on a perilous path in terms of diet, fitness, and emotional well-being? Someone you care about so much that you just want to shake them into making changes (with love, of course)? Maybe that someone is you? My colleague and friend, Dr. Craig Wax, also wants to shake you or your loved one awake, with loving concern, to regain a path of health, joy, light, and service.

Dr. Wax's book could not come at a better time, not only for your health journey, but for the entire country. Suddenly, there is a national movement to avoid toxins and find health. Why? It is because we have hit bottom, and we need warriors to fight back. For example, on a national level, there are shocking health statistics that must be reversed ASAP: 74% of Americans are dealing with overweight and obesity, 40% of children are dealing with the same, 52% of American adults suffer from prediabetes or Type 2 diabetes, 30% of teens have prediabetes, 1 in 31 children have autism, 34% of young adults have mental or behavioral disorders, early onset cancers have increased by 79%, 1 in 2 Americans are predicted to get cancer, autoimmune disease is rapidly rising, 18% of teens have fatty liver disease, 20-25% of women are on anti-depressant medications, low sperm count among men is an increasing concern, early onset dementia has tripled since 2013, American girls are starting puberty years earlier, infertility is rising rapidly, the highest infant mortality rate for a high income country, life expectancy on a decline, and, finally, 77% of young Americans are not able to qualify for military service. Is that enough?

I can relate to the passion with which Dr. Wax writes, as I have dedicated so much of my efforts to spreading the same messaging, admittedly, with a less edgy platform. I walked into the University of Michigan in 1977 as a timid, eighteen-year-old student, wondering why I had been accepted into a program where you started medical school right out of high school.

I was following Jewish dietary laws (kosher) and found the dormitory salad bar was the option that worked. That was the last time I ate animal foods because I realized how good I felt by limiting my diet to plant foods. My girlfriend, who was entering nursing school there, did the same, and she also noticed how good she felt. Fortunately, that salad bar led to a wedding and over 40 years of plant-based marriage to date.

As I studied medicine, I asked questions about nutrition that most students were not asking. I read articles and books outside my curriculum to gain more knowledge. During my cardiology fellowship training in the 1980s, a friend loaned me A Diet for a New America by John Robbins, and I started to understand a broader picture, including animal rights and the environmental issues addressed by a plant diet. Finally, just weeks after I began my cardiology practice back in Ann Arbor in 1990, Dean Ornish, MD, published the Lifestyle Heart trial, demonstrating that heart disease can be reversed through a plant-based diet, exercise, mind-body practices, and community. As this was pre-internet, I printed handouts for my patients to read on the ability of diet to prevent and reverse disease. Many read Dr. Ornish's best-selling book. When The China Study and other works were released, my patients were encouraged to read those too. Finally, the internet and documentaries like Forks Over Knives and others made it easy to teach patients in an efficient manner that food is truly medicine. The joy of having exposed thousands and thousands of patients to the idea that medication and procedures may not be necessary if they keep a laser focus on their diet and lifestyle, along with their mental well-being, has been so gratifying. Now I am excited to share this new book by Dr. Wax with them too.

Dr. Wax can teach you the power to avoid and heal what ails you, mentally, physically, or spiritually. Imagine a life less dependent on or completely free of medications, procedures, excess doctor visits, chronic pain, and disability – all by changing your mindset, changing your beliefs, eliminating your excuses, taking daily action, and upgrading the priority to feed your body premium nutrition for body and soul! Few have had the courage to speak the truth in the manner that Dr. Wax does. We owe him huge gratitude for charting the path and removing the obstacles. Now the decision is yours. Illness or health?

– Joel Kahn, MD, FACC
Clinical Professor of Medicine,
Wayne State University School of Medicine
Founder, Kahn Center for Cardiac Longevity
Triple board-certified

Award-winning author of multiple #1 bestsellers,
including *The Whole Heart Solution,*
Dead Execs Don't Get Bonuses,
The Plant-Based Solution, and *Lipoprotein(a)*

Recipient of awards from PETA and Crain's

Introduction

By Dr. Craig M. Wax

"The body has an innate intelligence that governs its every function."
– Andrew Taylor Still, DO

Ask yourself a few questions: Are we all living longer and healthier lives? Are you happy with your health and level of function? Are you satisfied with your weight and appearance? Do you eat #realfood? Is your primary drink plain water? With all the technology and interventions, are we truly leading better lives?

Congratulations on your commitment to learning how to improve and maximize your health. The so-called "holy grail" of health and disease is not a cure, but prevention. You make many investments in your life, but none is more important than the daily investment you make in your health. With the earned gift of health, you can achieve anything you set your mind to. Take responsibility, starting right now, and take the reins to guide your health to its fullest potential.

I wrote this book to explore the possibilities of achieving maximum health. If you ponder and then embrace its principles, you will be empowered to make healthy decisions. This is accomplished by helping you understand your body and its defenses, while also minimizing risks to your well-being. Lifestyle changes and health maximization techniques will be demonstrated. You will gain an understanding of your body, the stresses that work against it, and what you can do to thrive. It really is that simple.

The motivation to write this book began when I was an intern/first-year resident physician. I was in training at "The Heart Hospital." Daily, I diagnosed and treated cardiovascular disease according to the books and medical teachings. After listening to patients, understanding their lifestyle choices, I soon understood that a patient's lifestyle, primarily or secondarily, caused the disease. The poisons and toxins consumed, poor dietary choices, and lack of exercise contributed to their disease burden. I saw patients, prescribed potentially toxic chemical pharmaceutical meds, and sent patients for painful surgical procedures to "save" their lives. Conventional medicine practice, advocated for detection of established illness and prescribing many medications for secondary prevention, or to reduce their risk of a second heart attack or stroke. But what about primary prevention, or lowering a patient's risk of developing the disease process in the first place?

One morning, I was eating breakfast in the cafeteria of "The Heart Hospital," between ER admissions and making rounds, when I had a realization. I noticed that the hospital served sausage links and patties (fried meat), bacon (a more cured meat), "home fries" (fried potatoes), toast, and waffles (made from bleached white flour), as well as fried eggs, for breakfast. I watched as patients, their families, and hospital staff eagerly devoured their "food treats." It occurred to me that the hospital cafeteria's nutritional offerings were akin to dentists serving caramel and chocolate candy. Why did they serve this cardiovascular nightmare diet? The answer became clear: to sell food portions. The customers loved and regularly bought this "#notfood." These menu selections were driven by customer demand.

I began to ponder why consumers were demanding this toxic "#notfood." We'll explore my theory later—the Concentration-Stimulation theory.

Now, fast forward ten years. I attended an evening medical education conference, a "drug dinner," as they were commonly called. It was funded by a pharmaceutical company to educate physicians on the ravages of high cholesterol and implicitly tout their cholesterol lowering medication. This certain event was a steakhouse dinner lecture on cardiovascular disease. The speaker addressed one of its primary causes: hyperlipidemia (high and dysfunctional cholesterol) and diabetes mellitus (high and dysfunctional blood sugar). The doctor stated that patient lifestyle, poor diet, and lack of exercise were primary or secondary causes of cardiovascular disease. Other speakers discussed the challenges of getting patients to adopt a healthy diet, exercise, and lifestyle. The conversation quickly shifted to medical treatments, including expensive branded and potentially toxic drugs to improve the situation, or at least make it the "least worst," it could be if nothing else changed.

Then I looked around and saw my medical colleagues enjoying broiled and fried meats, fried potatoes, white flour bread products, and sugary desserts. "It was déjà vu all over again," to quote Yogi Berra. Had we learned nothing in ten years?

It became evident that not only had we failed to educate our patients, but we, as physicians, had also failed to change our own lifestyles and set a good example for health. At that moment that the drive to write this book became even more urgent.

On Independence of Thought

"The explorer for truth must first declare his independence. He must establish his observatory on hills of his own; he must establish it above the imaginary high planes of rulers, kings, professors of schools of all kinds and denominations. He must be the Czar of his own mental empire."

— Andrew Taylor Still, DO

Chapter One
Big Boy–The Fat Kid

"One gets large impressions in boyhood, sometimes, which he has to fight against all his life."

Mark Twain, *The Innocence Abroad*

Before I became a physician (doctor), I was a typical American child.

Growing up as a fat kid with two siblings, raised by two steadfast, working-class parents, taught me many lessons. We learned that sacrifice is necessary for the individual's and family's survival. My parents, primarily the children of immigrants themselves, sought to improve their circumstances and provide a better life for their children. Fortunately, they generated income from their commitment to work and raised children to meet their academic, religious, and moral standards. Unfortunately, a "better," life came with conveniences like fast-food #notfood.

Our family's journey encountered many challenges, and nothing came easily. Whatever we accomplished, we did it together, and it required dedication and consistency.

We accomplished moderate success, but it came with a price: obesity, which led to diabetes, cardiovascular disease, and an increased risk of colon cancer. Mom and Dad gained weight from their "luxury food," as Glenn Tilbrook of the British band

Squeeze called it, and the lack of formal exercise. We regularly ate fast food. Pizza, ice cream, cola/soda/pop, breaded fried chicken, and Philly soft pretzels were our first choices.

We considered cheese-steak, and "Italian Giant" subs a staple food (after all, my mom was from Philly, my father's sister ran a sub shop and catering business, and we lived in southern New Jersey near Philadelphia). We called them subs, but others called them hoagies, heroes, grinders, etc. All were the same—too much meat and cheese on white flour bread, and they always came with French fries – deep fat or oil-fried potatoes; starchy carbs in saturated fat!

Consequently, with all these #notfood items available in the house, I spent my childhood overweight and obese (and happy?).

Did you ever play the "reconsider game," of diminishing standards? I often did. While watching television (TV) or some other sedentary home activity, I would make the rounds of the kitchen, pantry, and cabinets, scrounging for a snack. It wasn't because I was hungry, but likely because I wanted the taste stimulation or I was just bored, or perhaps both(!). Anyway, I would make the rounds about every 15 minutes at TV commercial advertisement breaks to scavenge and turn up my nose at the lack of really desirable tasty snacks and mutter under my breath. Every time I made this voyage around the kitchen, stopping at the same places, picking up and putting down again the same items, my snack standards dropped a notch each time. Eventually, over time, I would make enough recurrent trips and drop standards enough notches to eat a worse item that I had no desire for or intention to eat in the first place. Have you ever played the reconsider game? If so, do you still play it?

The family called me "Big Boy" at home. I'm sure they meant it as a compliment somehow, but by my teenage years, it began to hurt. Neighborhood kids picked up on it, and it became mortifying. When they called me "Big Boy," I learned how to defend myself with humor, which motivated me to think critically about my life, try different strategies, make a plan, and take action.

Mom told me that an early moment of pride for her was that I took, not one, but two bottles of baby formula after my birth. Perhaps I would be healthy and grow big, but on artificial baby formula? Her doctor delivered me through a cesarean section surgery. In the 1960s, doctors told women that C-sections and fake baby formulas were better than natural vaginal deliveries and mothers' breast milk. Unknowingly, those doctors participated in mass media advertising propaganda espoused by industries that profited from the sale of surgeries and synthetic baby formulas. Today, doctors generally recommend vaginal deliveries unless there are complications. They encourage mothers to breastfeed, and these two modalities are generally considered the most physiologically and physically healthy options, as nature would have it.

Eating highly caloric, sugar, starch, and saturated fat-laden foods seemed normal to me as a child. Yet, despite my normal daily activities, my weight continued to climb. The Big Boy tag attached itself as early as grade school. It quickly became an insulting epithet that carried with it other stigmas when being chosen for sports teams. If a sport required running, the teams picked me last. They picked me first only for neighborhood sandlot football. They knew that when I took a handoff, I could barrel through the smaller, intimidated tacklers.

My size and body shape kept me warm in the winter, but I did sweat excessively in the summer due to my extra layers of abdominal adipose tissue, or fatty insulation (no, I did not know the term adipose at the time).

Buying school clothes left me mortified. In the 1970s, most northeastern moms took their kids to Sears (& Roebuck) and J.C. Penney's to buy new clothes for their children's continually growing bodies. My Mom, however, had no choice but to buy me "Husky Toughskins™ Corduroy" pants at Sears because nothing else would fit my expanded waist. Pulling them up on my large body felt like a disgrace; they were, indeed, "fat-boy pants." I was denied the immediate gratification of wearing the new clothes out of the store.

Nothing is more insulting than having to buy and wear "Husky Toughskins™ Corduroy" pants. Well, perhaps having a dad with a professional Singer sewing machine at work, hemming them up before you could even wear them, is just as insulting! But nothing could have been more insulting than when my schoolmates and neighborhood "friends" shared their daily honest observations with Big Boy and his fat-boy clothes.

Outwardly, children like me develop a good sense of humor as a defense mechanism to make kids laugh with me instead of at me. In my heart, it attacked my self-esteem and challenged me to build strong character.

At the time, there was no readily apparent information on ways to lose weight and get healthy. The only view I had of weight loss was the mom's dietary world of liquid protein bottles under the sink, thyroid meds, and prescription stimulants to reduce appetite and increase calorie utilization. For those averse to exercise (us!), there was even a passive movement center, mocking a gym. It featured machines that passively moved your limbs, likely accomplishing nothing.

I came to believe that my whole life would be that of an obese diabetic, like my mom. After all, I had learned somewhere along the way that genetics determined most outcomes. Wow, was I wrong (fortunately)!

Setback!

"Nobody told me there'd be days like these."

– John Lennon

Before I became a physician, alas, I was also a patient:

A week before leaving for college, now 18, while still living with my parents and siblings, I nearly lost my life. My friend asked me to go with him to look at a used car for sale. A Ford Mustang, a "muscle car" of the 1970s, set us off on what we hoped would be an exciting time, but not as "exciting" as it turned out.

A few days earlier, I had received a letter of acceptance to a college at a major university, where I planned to pursue a biology major, leading to a career as a physician. My life appeared to be on an upward trajectory.

On that misty, overcast afternoon, we drove to see the Mustang in my old (read: "classic") 1971 Chevy Malibu 350 V-8 (a "poor man's muscle car"). The car had a seat cover that covered up the seatbelt latches, meaning we never fastened them.

Going about 40 mph down a two-lane road, I readied myself to turn slightly as I approached an upcoming left bend. Then I saw, much to my horror, an oncoming car, a 1980 Cadillac (nicknamed "the tank") briefly appear and swing left in front of us, colliding with us head-on. Boom!

I don't remember the exact impact or the moments that followed. I may have lost consciousness. I do remember walking around the scene to look for my friend and surveying the wreck. My head bled from the top left, having made direct impact on the windshield and shattering it.

I felt numb all over and spaced out, in shock from the trauma. Fortunately, EMS had already arrived. Although I felt no pain, an EMT insisted that I wear a Philadelphia cervical collar to protect my neck; I reluctantly obliged.

"Where is my friend?" I asked. He sat motionless, still in the car. He had made facial contact with the dashboard—uh-oh! I thought surely, he would be admitted to the hospital, and I would be sent home. Wrong again!

The ambulance sped to a local hospital, and the EMTs took me into the emergency room. The medical staff quickly began their examination and ordered various tests, including blood tests, urine tests, X-rays, and a CAT scan. Someone called my parents (another uh-oh).

My friend had broken his nose and left foot. I still felt numb and dizzy but didn't feel the need to be fussed over. After all, I planned to drive to college in one week, but in what? The collision totaled my car.

X-rays and the CT scan showed I had broken my neck in two places. The terms meant nothing to me at first, but I quickly became familiar with them. The breaks had occurred at the "left side facet joint at C6-7 and the left transverse process of T1." This bad news shook me up. What is going to happen? I'm supposed to start school soon!

I recognized that if I took six months or a year to heal, I might never have started school. It would cost me the opportunity to achieve my lifelong goal of becoming a family physician. After orthopedic and spine consultations, I obeyed my doctors and followed a conservative course of therapy. My gracious parents and a wise guidance counselor helped me start college on time. I felt awkward wearing a Philadelphia cervical collar to school, certainly not a fashionable choice.

Freshmen commonly face academic challenges from the beginning. My challenges were also physical and emotional. Neck and back pain, with its dysfunction, became my constant companions. I felt it when I laid down to sleep and when I awoke in the morning, then all day long. I quit sleeping on my stomach because I couldn't breathe with my face pressed into the pillow. I tried to see myself as just another normal college teen but could not hide the neck brace nor mask my limited physical capabilities. The only pluses were the cafeteria ladies, who showed empathy and perhaps even pity for me and gave me extra food portions.

In addition to the first-year college curriculum, I made time for physical therapy sessions, to which I went two to three times a week. This included working with a therapist in his office and doing my daily home program. Looking back, I know I should have been more enthusiastic and dedicated.

A young man in college has multiple pursuits, many of which do not result in good health and longevity. I began to learn a lifetime lesson: one must be careful when testing and defining one's limits, or one could get derailed permanently.

Fortunately, I saw a spine surgeon at a prestigious hospital clinic in a nearby city. The surgeon was the brother of a local clothes merchant whom my dad knew, and whom we had patronized as children.

With my medical records, X-rays, MRIs, and consultation notes in tow, I headed to see the surgeon. (I learned another lesson: Parking is always a "joy" and too expensive.) Entering the surgeon's office, I checked in with the staff. A friendly but professional staff member handed me "oodles" of forms to complete.

After an hour or two, during which I tried to ignore my aches and pain, a nurse took me to the exam room where I met the orthopedic spine surgeon. He spoke kindly to me, telling me about his brother, the clothing merchant, who lived in our small, old town. We chatted about my life before and after the accident. He conducted a neurological and orthopedic spine exam.

After the exam, he explained that I wasn't a surgical candidate. "What about my daily pain?" I asked.

"You're a smart young man," he replied. "Get on with your life," after which he quickly left the room. The bad news left me frustrated and even mad. Who is he to tell me I would live with neck pain forever and just get on with life?!

I sat there for a bit, thinking that certainly, there must be something about the neck/spine that medical art and science can fix. They must be able to restore me to a healthy and pain-free life. I scheduled another consultation with a different neurosurgeon at a prestigious hospital in the city, hoping for a better outcome. How could it be worse? (PS: Never ask that question.)

I sat on the waiting list to be seen by this other spine surgeon at a major city university's "hand center" for six months. Time painfully dragged on, but I occupied myself doing the best I could in my classes.

Finally, the day came, and my parents took me to my appointment at the hand center. We were instructed to report to the clinic at 10:00 AM to complete the paperwork. (It was the mid-1980s. Doctors used paper medical charts, and no one had yet heard of the internet/web.) I wore my cervical collar and carried my insurance card, physical therapy reports, X-rays, MRIs, and we paid too much to park in the city garage. At any rate, pun intended, there we were.

We reported to the desk and received the salutary ream of paperwork. We sat down and, with pen in hand, began filling out the forms on the clipboard: a medical history form, a payment responsibility form, a privacy form, and what seemed like a dozen others.

Next, we sat and sat until noon. Was the surgeon in an emergency surgery or just running late for some reason? The desk staff instructed us to go to lunch across the street from the hospital and return by 1 PM. At this point, we were grateful for the break and went across the street for fast food (what else, but the staple of our daily diet?).

Not wanting to miss our appointment, we arrived back before 1 PM and checked in. More time passed. People came, saw the doctor, and left, but not us. My parents went to the counter a few times over the hours to inquire, but we were asked to return to our seats.

At 5 PM, the staff again engaged us and suggested that we

eat dinner, again, across from the medical center campus. Too mentally tired to question, we set off, this time to the Greek diner. Yet again, we returned early, so as not to miss our appointment. My parents again checked us back in at the desk by 6 PM for their evening session, although we had been scheduled for 10 AM.

I am unsure what time it was when, finally, a medical assistant took us to the exam room. How about 9 PM?! Here we four sat in a small 10x12 ft room where we saw an exam table, sink cabinetry, two chairs, and a rotating stool jammed inside the accordion door. It felt like a telephone booth, or an English phone box. (If you're born after 2000, look it up or watch an old rerun of "Doctor Who," the BBC UK science fiction series.)

At about 9:30 p.m., a chunky, balding, middle-aged man in scrubs (I'm not mincing words here), apparently the surgeon, entered the room. "Good evening," he said, with our charts under his arms. "Now, which one of you has neck pain?"

In that instant, I knew he hadn't read my chart or knew anything about my case. It made me angry. "Everyone in your damn waiting room has neck pain. We've waited for you for almost 12 hours, and that's after a 6-month wait for an appointment," I answered not so kindly.

With my chart still wedged under his arm, he asked, "Are we done then?"

"No, sir. We are not done!" I answered. "Sit down. Review my chart. Examine me, and let's be friends." He looked at me for a second and processed my statement.

He sat down at the sink, on the rotating stool. He showed us his back as he reviewed the chart. He then asked us a few clarifying questions about the history and my pain. He did a brief orthopedic and neurological exam. He concluded that I wasn't a surgical candidate. It left me stunned, again! How would I reduce my pain and be normal again or would that be impossible?

It took a while to process these consultations, my emotions, frustrations, concerns, and fears. It made no sense to me, a college freshman with his life before him. How could this be?

Today, looking back on the first orthopedic spine consultation, I understand it better now. The surgeon tried to tell me that life has its pains, and not all are fixable or even reducible. He told me that I am smart and had a bright future, but I HAD TO GET ON WITH IT. Now I know he had it right, although he needed practice on his bedside manner; a better choice of words was needed. I had to accept that I could never return to a pain-free state, but I could lead a gratifying life of meaning and joy.

From that devastating setback in my life, I learned some critically important lessons about living. Honestly, I don't know what the future holds for me and my health (no one does!), but I had the choice to adopt good health techniques and a healthy lifestyle to prepare for it, and to recover from life's setbacks and pitfalls.

Chapter Two
Common-Sense Revolution

"The body is a unit; a harmonious whole made up of mutually dependent parts."

–Andrew Taylor Still, DO

There is a new revolution in healthcare that, in fact, may not be so new: taking control of your health.

What if you took ownership of your health? This would (finally!) result in personal accountability and put you in control of your healthcare destiny. There is good news: It is possible. Remarkably, the process is neither difficult nor complicated. It requires a basic understanding of what goes on in your body and the forces that act upon it daily. The "magic" comes when you accept and understand this information and then use it to maximize your health. Does it sound complicated? It's not. This is the common-sense revolution, otherwise a revolution of common-sense.

A few centuries ago, the brightest minds thought and taught that evil spirits were responsible for sickness and death. This "fact" helped them explain what they could see but not understand. It provided a mechanism for what they observed. The early medical practitioners, "The Shaman" or "Medicine Man," relied on fear and superstition to explain the disease process. What did they believe or say about the health process?

Early medical practitioners like the Shaman or Medicine Man operated within spiritual, religious, and cultural frameworks, rather than scientific ones. They relied on fear and superstition largely because they didn't have access to biological or medical knowledge as we know it today.

Disease was considered the result of spiritual forces. Illness was often believed to be caused by evil spirits, curses, or the displeasure of gods or ancestors. Shamans might say a person got sick because they angered a spirit, violated a taboo, or were cursed by someone using magic.

Healing was a spiritual journey. Health was seen as a balance between body, mind, and spirit (Now we are getting somewhere!). Healing involved rituals, chants, herbal remedies, and communication with the spirit world, often in a trance or altered state.

Fear was a tool to control the masses of subjects. Shamans used fear to control behavior and maintain social order. For example, they might warn that breaking community rules would result in illness as punishment from the spirits.

At that time, they utilized superstition-based practices. Items like charms, amulets, or protective talismans were used to ward off disease. They might perform rituals to "extract" the evil or use smoke, drumming, or animal sacrifices to cleanse the body or space.

Health was a Reflection of Harmony between the spirit world and nature. Good health meant a person was in harmony with nature, spirits, and the community. Illness meant there was an imbalance—either internal (like guilt or spiritual impurity) or external (like a curse or attack).

So, in short, early shamans and medicine men explained disease through spiritual and supernatural causes, not biological ones. They believed healing required restoring spiritual balance, often through ritual and belief, not medical treatment in the modern sense.

Physicians and scientists have known for over a century that the body has a stake in its own health and a starring role to play in it. Despite all our technological advances, we remain in the dark about many bodily systems and processes. This makes the professional healthcare community very uncomfortable. Though we regularly make small advances that allow us to reduce pain and suffering and prolong life, we still must contend with the unknown.

We now see that we can partially halt a disease process with selective toxin medications; "robbing Peter to pay Paul," as it were. We can also partially reverse the course of coronary heart disease by using a major surgical operation to repair the heart. This involves cutting the rib cage open and stretching it, then stitching human-recycled or synthetic blood vessels around the heart. This should improve the heart's blood flow, but it is invasive, painful, expensive, and can subject the patient to the risk of stroke, infection, other complications, and death. It does nothing to change the causes of the disease that caused the heart trouble in the first place. So, is it really a solution?

The physician discovers heart disease (or any other disease for that matter) by examining a patient's family history, history of preexisting conditions, signs, and symptoms, and physical examinations. What if, however, instead of thinking in terms of the preexisting disease, the physician and patient considered prevention? What if individuals could make lifestyle changes many years before the disease presents itself, thereby preventing it? It is possible!

Conventional medical thought dwells upon the disease process. "Alternative medicine" practitioners advocate for various techniques to augment the body's defenses and maintain good health. The new common-sense revolution shares both views but emphasizes the empowerment and responsibility of everyone for their health.

There are times when sickness and conditions overwhelm the human body, and disease ensues. Common sense instructs us that everyone needs to achieve a healthy lifestyle through understanding our body's defenses and stresses. This common-sense revolution supports individuals in their goal to become healthy and stay healthy, and to recover more quickly when events occur that are beyond their control. Therefore, individuals feel better, perform better, get sick less often, and have a great sense of well-being.

Using this concept is easy and benefits everyone: individuals, their family, their workplace, and the government (yes, even the government stands to benefit. And, who funds the government? We ALL do…). So, come along and we'll see how the common-sense revolution can help you.

Health Insanity

This is a human paradox: We do all the wrong things (bad habits) every day and hope for an illogical healthy outcome. Our unhealthy lifestyle choices lead to sickness and death, yet we call upon other entities to save us from ourselves. "We are all just prisoners here, of our own device," from the song Hotel California by The Eagles. We expect participation from both private and public institutions, including insurance companies, the medical industry with its complex healthcare systems, and all levels of government, to help us maintain our health or recover from illness. This sort of hope can be destructive and terribly expensive. The right kind of hope is key to better health, but only if it motivates you to perform your daily health tasks more effectively, such as hydrating with water, eating a vegetable-based diet, and exercising regularly.

It is dangerous to you, and costly to everyone, to defer your choices and responsibilities to other entities. Insurance companies, hospitals, and the private medical industry will charge you a great deal of money to attempt to deliver you from the brink of disaster; the logical results of your unhealthy habits. Government entities try to tell you how you must live when they ban items or fine you for behaviors that they consider inappropriate or harmful. The government will take away your rights to interact with what it considers a problem. The real problem, however, is a lack of individual education, motivation, commitment and action.

When it comes to your health, there is only one person who cares, or should care. YOU are the only responsible entity and should be the only decision-maker in your affairs. (Sorry for shouting in all caps, but it's obvious that I am emphatic about it.)

What other entity or combination of outside forces can fix or prevent an individual's health problem? None. The only effective, efficient, and lasting solution is YOU! (There I go again, shouting about empowering the individual…) The good news is that you are uniquely qualified to solve your problems by making healthy choices. The bad news, if there is bad news, is that making healthy choices requires education, a positive attitude, decision making and discipline every day.

> We take pills to prevent the logical consequences of our choices and actions.
>
> We drink "not water." We eat "not food," #notfood.
>
> We do "not exercise." We do "not sleep.".
>
> We consume poisons. We take pills to eat. We take pills to drink.
>
> We take pills to sleep. We take pills to stay awake.
>
> We take pills to think. We take pills not to overthink.

We take pills to have sex. We take pills to avoid unpleasant feelings.

We take pills to treat the side effects of our other pills.

Does this sound like a dystopian novel? It is current reality, but it doesn't have to be your current reality.

Car maintenance vs body maintenance

"The body possesses self-regulatory, self-protective, and self-healing mechanisms."

–Andrew Taylor Still, DO

Most individuals have a basic understanding of owning and operating a car and what it requires. They know how to drive it, feed it gasoline, and may have a basic knowledge of how to maintain it.

Adults buy a car, usually with a car loan, and make interest and principal payments over four or five years. They find, or at least know, there is a detailed manual in the car to show them how to operate and maintain it. It helps the owner anticipate what to expect from the car. They can even take driving lessons to start or improve their techniques. Car owners also must obtain a driver's license to permit them to operate their cars on the roadways. Obtaining a license requires studying the driver's rule manual, passing a written and practical driving test, and paying a yearly fee for the privilege. Furthermore, they must register the vehicle with the state. This, too, requires an annual fee. States require all drivers to purchase car insurance to cover damage losses in accidents involving others. Auto insurance will also pay for basic personal injury care resulting from auto accidents. Last but not least, many states require periodic vehicle inspections to ensure vehicles are safe, sound to drive, and do not pollute the air more than the standards allow. These state requirements are fee-driven.

Meanwhile, a person drives their vehicle nearly every day for basic needs, such as shopping for clothes and food, commuting to work, and occasional pleasure trips. Despite the sure reality that cars are constantly depreciating in value, making them a poor investment, most people readily spend whatever time and money is needed. Cars, and how we use and care for them, have become staples of modern living across the developed world. Almost universally, all adults are familiar with and have paid for the above processes as they operate their cars daily.

Now, compare your car to your body; the only thing that you will always own.

What about the routine care and maintenance of the human body? Is there a user's manual for proper operation? Do you need a license to operate yours efficiently and sensibly? Must I take lessons? Is health insurance necessary for your pursuit of the best health and routine maintenance? Are you getting the full value and use out of the world's most incredible machine, your body? The answer to all these questions for most individuals is "no." You can, however, take lessons from your personal physician, nutritionist, physical therapist, personal trainer, chef, or other member of the healthcare team.

If people take good care of their cars, they can usually get at least 10 years' use out of them. What if I told you that, with proper education on the care and maintenance of the human body, you could potentially live 100 healthy years? Would you invest your resources, time, and best efforts to care for your ultimate investment: your body and its overall health? It sounds like a no-brainer, but, as we speak, it is most certainly not happening in the developed world. People readily take responsibility for the "health" and maintenance of their possessions, such as their cars, in order to get the maximum use, enjoyment, and "life" out of them. Why do they not do the same or better for their only true and lifelong possession, their body?

The Incredible Human Body

"I looked at the body and what did I find? I was in the presence of the most amazing machine ever conceived."

–Andrew Taylor Still, DO

The body is the most amazing automatic machine. It has the capacity for self-repair, physical activity, and mental calculations. It appreciates the arts and experiences an innate ability for emotion. No manmade machine can begin to approach the intricate simplicity and intrinsic wisdom of the human body. It embodies certain unalienable truths.

Despite the sometimes-overwhelming negative influences we encounter every day, can we achieve and maintain good health? What can be done "to take arms against a sea of troubles?" as Shakespeare questions in Hamlet, "…and by opposing, end them." The answer is to accept responsibility for the knowledge of good health habits and then use them to your advantage.

The body is endowed with intrinsic wisdom, healing power, and incredible self-maintenance powers. Voltaire said. "*Medicus curat, natura sanat.*" "The job of the physician is to amuse the patient while nature cures the disease." This refers to the body's innate abilities and the historical doctors' inability to understand the intrinsic wisdom of the body.

The more we study the human body, the more questions that remain. We can, however, do more than merely marvel at nature. We can devote our minds to understanding it, and work with our bodies to become the fullest expression of humankind, that is, having good health.

"*Seek health, it enables all things*," Craig M. Wax, DO.

The human body, mind, and spirit possess self-regulatory processes. It has a built-in pharmacy that supplies hormones, neurotransmitters, and other natural chemicals to facilitate billions of reactions and processes every second. Every cell functions as part of a larger unit, synchronously and in concert with every other cell. Cells are organized into functional tissues called organs. These autonomous organs are integrated into organ systems; all are governed by the feedback and orders of the neurological and endocrine systems, with the brain at the top of the command chain. This enables the human body to function as a coordinated whole.

Technology brings us ever closer to the smaller and smaller functional units within individual cells. Each part does its job to support the greater whole. Each time we gain a closer look, we are amazed to find yet smaller units functioning on an intelligent but basic level. These small sub-cellular and even sub-atomic parts never rest. They work day and night to nourish and advance the causes of the whole organism, the whole body, which we call human "life."

Chapter Three
The Osteopathic Approach

"To find health should be the object of the doctor. Anyone can find disease."

— Andrew Taylor Still, DO

In the 1850s, Andrew Taylor Still (1828-1917) became a Medical Doctor (MD) trained in the traditional methods of his day. Dr. Still's original MD medical studies included scholastic work but primarily consisted of apprenticeship with practicing physicians. This type of learning produced trained doctors who became known as Medical Doctors, or MDs.

By 1874, as a conventionally trained MD allopathic physician, Dr. Still had become frustrated with the traditional medicine of his day. It alarmed him that those doctors relied too often on treating patients with poisonous heavy metal "medicines." He knew there had to be a better way to approach patient care.

It wasn't until 1874 that he "flung the flag of Osteopathy to the breeze," becoming the first American Osteopathic Physician. Later, after years of practice, he started the American School of Osteopathy in Kirksville, Missouri, in 1892.

Dr. Still began to practice Osteopathic medicine. He saw it as a discipline that met a wide range of patient needs. It relies on a health maintenance philosophy that incorporates "hands-on" techniques to remove impediments to health, alleviate pain, and speed healing. As a hunter and anatomist, he had acquired a vast knowledge of anatomy and human physiological functions. He came at his practice with an open mind, applying the good he had learned from medical training and serving patients to create a new school of medicine. This became known as a Doctor of Osteopathy: DO.

Today, American DOs are fully trained and licensed medical physicians in all states. They receive equivalent training to MDs and receive additional training in a holistic wellness approach and hands-on physical manual medicine. They practice in all specialty areas of training. They are most well-known, however, for their comprehensive family medicine and other primary care specialties, like internal medicine, pediatrics, and gynecology. "The role of the osteopath is to help the body help itself," said Dr. Still.

The DO's medical and surgical training is augmented by a unified, holistic philosophy that treats the whole person. In addition to conventional training, they receive extensive instruction on osteopathic principles and practices (OPP) and osteopathic manipulative treatment (OMT) techniques. OMT is now called Osteopathic Manual Medicine (OMM). OMM includes soft tissue stretching techniques related to deep massage, muscle energy resistance techniques similar to those used in physical therapy, and thrusting techniques similar to those used in chiropractic care. Interestingly, Daniel David (D.D.) Palmer, himself a magnetic healer who went to the early American School of Osteopathy, never finished his studies. He left to start the first Chiropractic school, as the story goes. This Osteopathic comprehensive approach predates both chiropractic and physical therapy.

Hands-on techniques, remarkably, are nothing new. "Healers" have used them for centuries throughout the world with much success.

Osteopathic philosophy is based on a common-sense approach to health. It maintains that, if properly cared for, the body can grow, heal, and thrive. This concept can be broken down into simple postulates per Dr. Still's teachings, practice, and writings.

The body is a unit. All the organs work together to provide the body with its functionality. This includes the muscles, bones, nerves, digestive tract, and the brain. They work in harmony with producing and maintaining health. No organ can properly function separately from the others, as "no man is an island." It is for this fundamental reason that the physician and patient must treat the whole body; no part is separable from the rest.

The body possesses self-regulatory mechanisms. All body systems have feedback mechanisms to ensure their proper performance. Consider controlling blood sugar. Glucose is a sugar that is necessary to produce energy in a cell. Therefore, the glucose levels must be carefully maintained. Too much glucose can cause damage to the small blood vessels. This destruction of small blood vessels can lead to blindness and kidney failure, as well as heart attacks, strokes, and other life-threatening health maladies. Too little glucose leads to the starvation and death of cells all over the body.

Your body obtains glucose from the food you eat. It is absorbed in the gastrointestinal tract. The body uses some of that glucose immediately to fuel essential bodily processes and stores the excess as fat.

Hormones, such as insulin, regulate the use and uptake of sugar. Insulin is produced in the pancreas and transported through the blood, alongside absorbed glucose.

Insulin is critical for glucose absorption in body tissues. Without sufficient functional insulin, the body cannot effectively handle the excess glucose, and diabetes mellitus ensues. Less commonly, with too much insulin, the body cannot accurately regulate glucose uptake. In this way, insulin production and utilization ensure that the body has enough energy to function and to store "for a rainy day." The brain oversees the absorption and use of glucose and other processes to provide a double check to ensure that the body is functioning correctly.

The arteries' role is critical. This is a poetic yet straightforward way to bring up the importance of a good, strong blood supply. Fresh, life-giving blood is one of the most urgent needs of every tissue in your body. It brings oxygen and nutrients to the body while removing impurities and waste products for disposal. If the arteries, capillaries, or veins are obstructed by plaque, disease, or toxins, the healthy blood supply slows and may even stop. Doctors call this vascular disease.

Vascular disease is to be taken seriously; it can cause the death of organs like the heart (cardiovascular disease) and eventually, death. This disease process should be avoided at all costs. The cost of good health is the reason for the common-sense revolution.

"Structure and function are intimately related." Anatomy is the study of the human structure and its components. Physiology is the study of tissue function. Dr. Still remained, first and foremost, an anatomist. He applied his understanding of the human body to the DO practice of medicine. He saw that the body is comprised of individual cells organized into tissues, organs, and organ systems that all work together. As they are so structured, so shall they function.

Organs are anatomically designed to function in specific ways. If they are structured correctly and well-maintained, they can work in peace and harmony. If a genetic malfunction causes organs to be incorrectly assembled at birth, or they develop poor structure due to disease, then they cannot function as intended. Good anatomical structure is vital to the proper functioning and maintenance of a healthy body.

Dr. Still is credited as the first physician to recognize the importance of fascia connective tissue for maintaining body health. Fascia governs not only the structure and range of motion but also the blood, lymphatic fluid, and interstitial fluid that flows throughout the body. This is critical to the metabolic process that must remove "trash" and bring in nutrients to nourish the cells.

Dr. Still's quote, "The rule of the artery is supreme," emphasizes the importance of proper blood flow for health, suggesting that when blood and lymphatic circulation are unobstructed, tissues can function optimally. This principle is foundational in osteopathy, highlighting the relationship between circulation and overall well-being.

Osteopathic medicine treats the body as a unified whole and the person as a unique individual. Each body part is related to the others and must be treated in conjunction with all of them. Each person needs to have their physical and emotional needs met to treat their illness and maintain their overall health effectively.

It is with accepted medical techniques and a hands-on approach that a Doctor of Osteopathic Medicine (DO) treats each person. These may include Osteopathic Manipulative Treatment (OMT), also known as Osteopathic Manual Medicine (OMM), medications, trigger point injection, surgery, exercises, diet, and always, nutrition counseling. It is through this comprehensive care that a person can recover and maintain good health for a lifetime.

Today's DOs practice comprehensive healthcare in the office, home, surgical center, and the hospital. They use a preventive approach and osteopathic manual medicine techniques to address everybody's needs.

Chapter Four
Bug vs Body (Germ vs Terrain)

"The doctor of the future will give no medicine, but will interest his patients in the care of the human frame."

– Andrew Taylor Still, DO

In general, people are familiar with the Twentieth Century's preoccupation and direction in medicine toward the germ theory. They observe that prions, viruses, bacteria, fungi, and other pathogens enter the body and cause disturbances and infections. We recognize that our body has a simple first line of defense, commonly called skin, to protect us. We know that there are more complex defenses, such as the immune system, to fend off and fight incoming infections, kill and remove mutant cancer cells before they grow and spread.

Physicians learn to diagnose infections and prescribe selective poisons, commonly known as antibiotics to kill the "bugs." But far too many ignore the body's innate defenses that stand against and defeat disease, and that help produce good health.

In the 1800s, two schools of thought emerged among scientists and physicians of the time regarding the understanding of disease. These came after the "evil spirits," and demonic possessions were largely disproven and rejected. A remnant that remains from this time is when a person reflexively says, "G-d bless you," after a sneeze. Initially, people said this out of fear that the devil would jump down their throat and wreak havoc on their health each time they sneezed. In the present day, obviously, this is not true, but it is still considered common courtesy to say, "Bless you," immediately after someone sneezes.

One school of thought explored the microbe (germ) theory, championed by Louis Pasteur. A second school of thought was Antoine Bechamp, who championed a cellular terrain theory. The microbe theory held that the bug caused illness and must be eliminated. The terrain theory held that the terrain, or body, must be resistant to bugs and other disease entities.

Andrew Taylor Still, DO, believed, and saw evidence that the medications of his time, like arsenic, mercury, and opium, were toxic. He further believed that vomiting, blistering, and bleeding patients, which were standard medical therapies in the 1800s, weakened and killed patients. He observed that as the body returned to its natural, normal order, it also returned to normal function, thereby preventing disease. He saw that structure and function are interrelated. To Dr. Still, the key element in helping a patient is to remove muscular, skeletal, nervous, and fluid flow restrictions through hands-on diagnosis and manual therapy. This allowed the body to return to resilience. Dr. Still's theories and hypotheses have withstood the test of time, from the Influenza epidemic of 1914 through the present day.

Over recent centuries, we have learned through science, research, medical practice, and physician experience that, although all play key roles, prevention strategies — based on improving the body's innate health and disease resistance — are the key that every individual holds in their hands.

In Pandemics, the elderly, frail, disabled, obese, ill, or otherwise immune-compromised individuals and populations are generally the most widely affected by morbidity and mortality from the bug or disease in question. Here is where you come in, at whatever age you are RIGHT NOW. You can maximize your health through a successful lifestyle, regular body monitoring, and making wise, effective changes. If you are young, start now. If you are middle-aged, time is a-wasting. If you are old, what are you waiting for? The clock will run out, and the mountain will win eventually, every time.

If you are a parent, you are the best teacher that your children will ever have. Babies, children, and even teens learn by watching what their parents say and do; more by what they do than what they say. Children, especially teens, will seem not to listen to you, but they will watch, learn, and emulate some of your behaviors and actions. Doing the right thing every day is better than saying the right thing.

It behooves all of us, whether we have children or not, to be a good example for the family we love, the friends we care about, and all others who look up to us. Believe it or not, it is even more important for physicians, nurses, therapists, and other healthcare practitioners to model the best behaviors. It is both healthy for us and instills confidence in our patients that we practice good health so that they can trust us with their health.

"It's a great day, isn't it?" I'll say when I greet a patient. "I rode 20 miles at dawn this morning outside on my recumbent bicycle." Next, I ask, "What are you up to?"

These questions are asked to let the patient know that I believe in and practice what I recommend to them. My words, actions, and questions help me engage and challenge them to practice and report healthy behaviors.

Genetic influence

Genetics plays a principal role in our bodies; in ourselves. Conditions and ailments do "run in our families." Yet, does this mean we are likely to face the same or similar health challenges as our parents and their siblings did?

If you are a woman whose mother had breast cancer, you

are also at a greater risk than someone with no family history of it. If you are a male whose brother and father died of a myocardial infarction or "heart attack," you are also at increased risk. These examples are true, but they are not the entire answer.

Recent studies suggest that lifestyle and dietary choices can influence genetic expression. It turns out that you have more control over your daily and lifelong health than you think.

You could say that your genes serve as a blueprint or building plan for your body, from your traits as a baby to your appearance and how you function on your final day. Your body sheds skin cells constantly, and it may even play a part in whether you are a morning or late-night person. Family history, or the medical conditions that seem to run in our families, can also play a significant role in our lives.

Genes and DNA determine the amount of functional reserve we have in each organ of our body. We are naturally endowed with an abundance of extra cells and functional tissue in each organ. For instance, if you need 50% of your lungs to survive, we have been given 100%: 50% over and above the 50% necessary to sustain life. This additional 50% is referred to as functional reserve. This ensures that there is plenty of room for learning and errors (lucky for us!). Most organs and body systems enjoy double the functional tissue that we actually need to survive. Each person has a different set of genes, and we all have different amounts of functional reserve. This explains why "Aunt Bessie" smoked cigarettes and lived to 90 and why "Uncle Irving" had a heart attack at age 40 and died of lung cancer at 60. "Uncle Irving" obviously had less relative functional reserve.

Genes may confer an individual risk for causing diabetes, hypertension, cancer, and other diseases. This is known as a genetic predisposition, and it is what makes family history so important.

Environmental risk factors also play a role. These are the behaviors, habits, and lifestyle choices that impact your body and health and can influence your genetic predisposition. Lifestyle choices can make it more or less likely for a gene to express itself. If your genes predispose you to diabetes, environmental factors will influence that outcome. If you weigh too much, eat sugar-laden foods, or do not exercise enough, you may indirectly cause your body to develop diabetes. This is a direct or indirect result of the decisions that you make every day! Wow, our choices about how we live are critical, even life-controlling.

In the 2000s, medical research produced relatively inexpensive "over the counter (OTC)" genetic testing kits. People can purchase these kits to take to a lab and have their genetic code analyzed. This is a good/bad thing or a bad/good thing, depending on circumstances, philosophy, and motivation.

The most personal thing a person owns is their unique genetic code, which is distinct from that of all others. This information may have value to you, but it can also be valuable to others. Genetic information, in aggregate, can be used to help prevent and cure diseases. Having said that, more frequently, your information can be stolen, bought, and sold, ultimately violating your most sacred right to privacy, genetic privacy. "Too many times privacy issues get ignored in the rush to make policy... the medical privacy and personal autonomy issues surrounding genetic research..." The genetic information, once sequenced and decoded in a lab, can be used for nefarious purposes, like biological targeting and warfare.

As you consider whether to have your DNA analyzed, consider why you are doing it. What is the reason you want this information? If you know that others may obtain and use it, ask yourself these questions:

1. Will you use the information?
2. How will you use the information?
3. With whom will you share the information?

4. How will you and your assignees keep information safe, private, and secure?

Physicians, nurses, and educators often fail to mention that environmental risk factors come into play. For instance, if a man lives a healthy lifestyle, but his father and brother did not, it is a significant part of why the young man never suffered from those "family conditions." The genetic influence is probably there, but an unhealthy lifestyle increases the risk of acquiring the disease. You have control over what you have control over, so why not minimize your risk factors? Then you will maximize your functional reserve. This will help decrease the likelihood of developing a health problem while maintaining good health.

Having said all that about genetic risks, the reality is that genes aren't even half of it. Prior to 1990, medical science taught that about 80% of health outcomes are determined by gene expression and about 20% by lifestyle, diet, and exercise choices. After 1990, it gradually became clearer that medical science had it backward. In truth, everyday lifestyle choices determine 80% of our outcomes, and genetics about 20%. What a difference time and experience makes!

Stress

Stress is undue pressure on the body's systems that affects its ability to perform its everyday duties. It forces the body to work harder to compensate for the extra pressure. Many outside influences can cause stress: job, home, relationships, emotional loss, taxes (on or about April 15!), toxins, poor diet, lack of exercise; just about everything, it seems!

My mother used to say, "stress kills," as she pointed, for effect, with a lit cigarette in her hand (Salem "lights"). Her action is both ironic and darkly humorous. She held a known poison and toxin generator in her hand and volitionally sucked it into her lungs and whole body in a dysfunctional response to life stressors. "Bad habits," like smoking tobacco and cannabis, drinking alcohol, and consuming other drugs and dangerous substances, worsen your health and lessen your resistance to stress.

Humans experience stress in various forms every day. Think of having a short temper, feeling pain, depression, changes in sleep, and countless others. Stress is a messenger telling us that our mind and body are having a tough time dealing with something. We must be vigilant and attentive to these signs, making them useful to restore or attain better health.

The good news is that the body is a great compensator and can cope with short bursts of stress. You can stay up late to finish a project and still work or attend school the next day. If you struggle to cope with temporary stress, it can become your constant companion. It will "nag" you into poor health. Coping with stress becomes increasingly challenging as we age. Our tissues become much thinner and work more slowly. It is vital to learn healthy ways to use stress for its intended purpose as a warning and then break free from it to maintain better health. When detected, it is very much like your car's "check engine" light on your dashboard. It informs you that something is amiss and requires attention. In your car, it may be anything from an insignificant loose gas cap to a quite significant oil leak, threatening the engine altogether.

Being in touch with your body means a person must develop their ability to "listen." This means employing all of the senses to "listen" to the body. You can feel when your breathing and heart rate quicken. This can occur in response to exercise, mental stress, or physical stress, or it may be the result of an infection or an underlying health challenge. We must be in tune with our body's signals and interpret them. No one gets this right 100% of the time, but each of us can learn to identify a stressor and better cope with it, thereby reducing its negative effects on our health.

Consider an argument you may have with a friend or family member. The mind-body connection is at work. Your heart rate quickens, and your breathing becomes more rapid. Your temperature may rise slightly. Your body begins to sweat to dissipate the heat. These are signs of the increased sympathetic nervous system doing its job. It is called the "fight or flight response." Over the eons of our existence, it has helped keep humans safe from invaders or animal attacks when threatened. The invader may be external, like a human enemy, or internal, like a virus or bacteria.

"In an emergency, first take your own pulse" is from the classic medical novel *The House of God* (1978), by Samuel Shem, MD. This line is one of the many darkly humorous "Laws of the House of God" shared in the book. It means that in a crisis, especially in medicine, the first thing a doctor should do is stay calm, not panic, so they can think clearly and act effectively. It is no different for anyone in a stressful situation. In fact, this book was one of my inspirations to become a physician, as it told the story of medical internship. The characters were three-dimensional, caring, and all too human. It was my privilege, in 2018, to give a presentation at the "Patient-Physician Association Conference," in Atlantic City, NJ, with Dr. Shem as the keynote speaker. When I presented his quote to the audience, everyone understood its message, and he was gratified and honored.

If we are aware of these physical and mental messages, we can adjust our response to the stressor. In doing so and "calming down," we will minimize the damage that stress does to our system. This is why it is essential to understand the importance of feelings, thoughts, and relationships in our daily lives.

In any stressful situation, there is a transmitter. This is a word, deed, or article that could cause a dystonic or unpleasant feeling in the receiver. The receiver tunes into it and responds with stressful sympathetic nervous response. Sometimes the reaction is automatic. However, in most situations, if the intended receiver is in tune with his/her body, to their thoughts and feelings, they can sense that the stress may escalate. Once detected and understood, the receiver can choose not to initiate the sympathetic nervous system response. This is crucial to prolonging the quality and longevity of the body, mind, and spirit. Breathwork, meditation and yoga are excellent practices for connecting with your body's intrinsic rhythms and reducing stress.

How can mud be the stressor? What if, while you stand innocently by, someone throws a handful of mud at you? Quick! What do you do? There are three options: 1) Let the mud hit you. 2) Throw mud back at the other person. 3) Duck and let the mud sail past you. You might also choose to run away, fast.

If the mud hits you, chances are that your body will respond to the stress by increasing your sympathetic tone. You will get "worked up" and experience feelings of upset, anxiety, fear, or anger. This may lead you to throw mud back, an acceptance of the conflict state. It creates a state that makes your body vulnerable.

If you duck and let the mud whiz by, you are not validating the conflict. You may feel the urge to respond with righteous anger, but it's actually more energy-efficient. You conserve your personal resources so you can use them more efficiently, calmly, and in a rational mental state. This efficiency and life force conservation will enable you to increase your natural defenses against invaders that you may not be so quick to detect, those that will sneak up and attack you from behind. This is the basic concept described in The Sedona Method, by Hale Dwoskin.

Indeed, we cannot end all stress. However, we can minimize stress and its adverse effects on our bodies. The keywords here are prevention and healthy lifestyle.

Prevention entails "plugging in" to the causes of stress and being alert to our responses to them. Perhaps we can begin to work fewer hours at a time, or, if not, work more efficiently. This means taking occasional short breaks to get some water or stretch our muscles. This allows for better circulation and enables the mind to refocus on the task at hand.

Better planning of work and projects reduces stress associated with meeting deadlines. It's a simple yet straightforward idea that pays off in reduced stress as a deadline approaches.

A later chapter summarizes a healthy lifestyle. A few key requirements include avoiding toxins, following a low-saturated fat and cholesterol diet with high fiber and plant protein, engaging in daily exercise, maintaining a regular sleep pattern, and fostering healthy relationships. These are all essential for maximizing the body's health and its ability to handle the stress of daily living.

Chapter Five
Why Are We Failing On All Fronts?

"Failure isn't fatal, but failure to change might be."

– John Wooden

Viewed as a total society in our "modern, developed country," the United States population is failing miserably when it comes to their wellness lifestyle, health, and healthcare. Please note the differences. Wellness lifestyle refers to your daily activities, maintenance, and self-care. Health is your current, ever-changing state of well-being. Healthcare includes medical, surgical, alternative, and emergency professional care that we access. We spend more than any other developed nation on healthcare services, tests, procedures, and our mostly feeble attempts to improve our health. The combined spending on healthcare, health insurance, government public health programs, and other related expenses has not resulted in better health.

Those with private health insurance see their premiums spiraling higher each day and increases in government regulation and the rapid evolution of medical care make the delivery of healthcare services more challenging (they are directly related). By any fair standard, however, we seem to finish near the bottom in terms of good health outcomes and longevity. We also have huge individual and government debt, potentially beyond repayment if present trends continue.

What do the primitive survival aspects of our brain chemistry beckon us to do? We steal food, money, gamble, and commit "crimes of passion" to satisfy intense wants. Some turn to legal drugs like tobacco, alcohol, cannabis (legal in some states), caffeine, saturated animal fat, and table sugar. Others turn to illegal or illicit drugs that become cycles of deadly habits, ultimately causing sickness and death. These destructive practices all have a common thread: humans like and want stimulation at every waking moment. We desire it. We crave it. We will do anything to get it. Stimulation, whether by food, chemicals, toxins, physical contact, video screens and devices that bombard our senses, loud music, or by any other means, has become vital to human existence and enjoyment.

Just why are we predominantly overweight and becoming more obese, putting our health at risk for failure? One reason is that our lives are unnecessarily complicated due to an increasing number of time-consuming tasks. This results in less time for meals and fewer meals per day.

After our nightly sleep, we wake dehydrated and ready to take in water and a balanced, nutrient-dense, vegetable-based meal called breakfast, literally breaking the normal nightly fast. This is why nutrition experts and health advocates stress the importance of a healthy breakfast meal and, even more importantly, adequate water intake to start your day off right.

We need food to survive, such as vegetables, whole grains, fruit, and fish, but bombard ourselves with ultra-concentrated food derivatives (#notfood, as I call them), including candy, cake, ice cream, cheese, white bread, pasta, soft drinks, alcoholic beverages, etc. These are not foods made by nature, but by people for sale to people for profit. Daily, we select concentrated food derivatives due to our nature to survive.

Since the beginning of humanity, real food (#realfood, this time affectionately) has come, and continues to come, from the Earth through natural processes, such as organic farming. Now, through chemistry labs, factories, "big food" agribusiness, and the meat industry, we are presented with super-concentrated or synthesized food-like products that appeal to our most basic sense of survival. So, why is our survival instinct killing us with obesity, diabetes, vascular disease, strokes, and heart attacks? Oh, cancer… I can't forget to mention cancer. That's a biggie.

The leading causes of death in the U.S., as of 2023, are heart disease, cancer, accidental injuries, stroke/cerebrovascular disease, COPD/Chronic lower respiratory disease, Alzheimer/dementia, diabetes, kidney disease and cirrhosis/chronic liver disease. This list is in descending order, compiled and published by the Centers for Disease Control (https://www.cdc.gov/nchs/fastats/leading-causes-of-death.htm).

Humans are meant to go through natural cycles of feast and famine. In the developed world's supermarkets, there is no such thing as famine, only super-concentrated feasting for all shoppers, every hour, and every day. When humans instead consume chemical pharmaceutical poisons, they become rotund, obese, and sickly. To continue their existence, they turn to modern medicine, paying whatever it costs for more miserable, sickly days, months, and years of life. It is a sad scene.

We have a fantastic human body that can self-maintain and self-regulate. In today's mentally stressful work-world, while consuming food-concentrate-derivative products sold in our supermarkets, fast-food joints, and online, we have become a pitiful bunch of individuals! Were it not for expensive, toxic medications and expensive, painful, and often debilitating surgical procedures, we would die prematurely of preventable illness. Or must we?

Concentration/Stimulation Theory

Why are all developed countries rife with massive obesity and related diseases running rampant among their populations? Why do humans in developed countries eat super-concentrated imitation food derivatives? Why can't we seem to control our dietary intake to produce lean and fit people? Ah, all good questions. I believe the answer to all three is "concentration and stimulation." The concentration of calories from saturated fat and sugar in super-concentrated food derivatives, as we consume them, leads to weight gain, obesity, and disease. Why are we failing now when we succeeded in surviving thousands, if not millions, of years? Life is a game of expectations. It's not rocket science, but rather neuroscience, involving neurotransmitters, notably dopamine and norepinephrine.

Concentration

Concentration refers to the number of particles (solute) per unit of liquid (solvent). The primary biological solvent is water. Naturally grown foods like vegetables and fruits tend to be much less concentrated with particles than so-called processed foods. Cheese, ice cream, and butter, for example, although the dairy industry and USDA (the government self-designated police and marketing arm), consider them "processed foods," are not food at all. That's right, they do not pass the litmus test for food. All real food must be in natural concentration as it occurs in the environment. There is nowhere on Earth, not even a farm, which has a block of cheese, a gallon of ice cream, or a pound of butter sitting on the grass, waiting to be picked. They are all derived from natural foods that have been super concentrated to become food derivatives that, when eaten, overwhelm your gastrointestinal and nervous systems with their ultra-high concentration. They are so concentrated in calorie density and saturated fat, cholesterol, salt, sugar, and other particles that trigger your brain and body to store the excess calories as fat in your body. Our bodies cannot handle large portions of super-concentrated food derivatives.

People in the U.S. and other developed countries have a food industry that seeks to profit from selling highly concentrated food derivatives. Please understand that I am an advocate for free market competition and business for profit. Ralph Waldo Emerson's concept, "Build a better mousetrap, and the world will beat a path to your door," is a metaphor for this. My primary concern is of those people and entities selling ultra-concentrated #notfood, poisons, and toxins. Individuals struggle to control their impulses to eat these products because they are influenced by both nature and nurture. We constantly subconsciously take in advertisements for these items on the radio, TV, computers, and the internet. We are super-saturated with ads during most of our waking moments.

The immigrant from a poor, foreign nation stands in shock the first time he or she enters one of our modern supermarkets. Such abundance! Such a number of choices! They are unaware that the supermarket is stocked with 80% super-concentrated food derivatives and formulated products that, over time, will damage their bodies. It seems to be a challenge to find #realfood.

"From 2008 to 2010, children's and teens' exposure to television ads for soda doubled, according to a report from the Rudd Center for Food Policy & Obesity at Yale University. And, beverage companies targeted black and Hispanic kids more than others in recent ads, the report found. Commercials for Coke and Dr. Pepper products led the increase."

Sucrose, or "table sugar," as it is commonly known, is also a concentrated #notfood. The big-food sugar industry has found its way deep into the American psyche, our brains, and our bodies. In fact, they've labeled it "table sugar" to make you believe that it belongs on your kitchen table! Think about that for a second. It was a hugely successful marketing and advertising campaign. Still today, the industry and government entities advertise table sugar as natural.

Soda, pop, and cola beverages have been extremely popular over the last 100 years. They appeal to one's "sweet tooth." Sodas have ten teaspoons of sugar in just a twelve-ounce serving. "One soda a day equals 50 pounds of table sugar (sucrose) a year." This is a very concentrated sugar load for the body to handle. The body must dilute it with water and produce more insulin to deal with the sugar. Sodas also contain phosphoric acid and caffeine; both can irritate the stomach. Caffeine is also the stimulant chemical to lift you out of your sugar crash that sodas cause. Originally, Coca-Cola had cocaine in it, while 7-Up had lithium in it. Look it up. It is history. Caramel coloring, a mess of chemical reaction compounds and sugar, which both add to cola's taste and color, stains and decays the teeth, causes diabetes, and even cancer. We all should eliminate these beverages from our diet.

The keystone to our U.S. and world obesity epidemic is our innate body programming, in my opinion. Our bodies are designed to exercise, drink water, and eat natural foods that come from the Earth. However, the last 100 years of exponential obesity growth teach us that, when given the choice between broccoli and a candy bar, most will choose the candy bar. Why? Again, concentration/simulation is the reason, but each individual is responsible.

Throughout human existence, the body hasn't always had unfettered access to food. There have been droughts, floods, an inability to farm or hunt, and adverse weather conditions, among other challenges. Our body is innately pre-programmed to survive. This is achieved by consuming calories when available in a grazing manner, similar to how cows do it.

To survive, our body craves the highest concentration of calorie-dense foods available. Before the Industrial Revolution, this wasn't a problem; mostly, only natural foods were available well into the 1800s. In the twentieth century, "food" producers created an industry selling us refined, non-food super-concentrated food derivatives. Since our bodies crave calories to survive, the "food" industry prospered, earning a massive profit, convincing us not only that their "food" is good for us, but also that it brings pleasure to life. Unfortunately, this has expanded the obesity epidemic beyond previous projections to encompass half the population of the U.S. by 2030. According to the Centers for Disease Control, we are well on our way to that unfortunate "goal."

Approximately 40.3% of U.S. adults by 2023 were considered obese." And the rest of the developed world is following our lead.

Do not buy into society's, government's, or marketing views of what your diet should be. Whenever possible, opt for natural foods found on Earth and drink water; these are always the best choices. If what catches your attention only comes in a can, Mylar™ bag, box, or bottle, it likely isn't food for a healthy body.

Stimulation

Our central nervous systems crave stimulation that results in the release of neurotransmitters like dopamine, which stimulates our pleasure centers. These can lead to enhanced survival and reproduction, but in our artificial, unnatural, human-made environment, they lead to obesity, disease, addiction, and death.

Our brains crave stimulation that most of us find in concentrated calorie-enhanced food derivatives. We are intrinsically motivated to believe that these foods contribute to power in our lives, fostering pleasurable interpersonal relationships and improved sex. Supported by media stimulation, we spend lavishly on unhealthy food, objects, and services. This, however, can lead to dependency and addiction.

The good news is that we do not have to be slaves to government, media, big money and material possessions, big food corporations, the toxin stimulant industries like tobacco, alcohol, caffeine, and power brokers in our society. We can choose to be stimulated by healthy natural food from the Earth, daily exercise, healthy human relationships, and self-confidence and resilience that come from the achievement and maintenance of one's health.

Have you ever noticed that we tend to devour our food quickly, taking increasingly larger bites or gulps? Why? The answer is simple. We are programmed by nature to enjoy and seek stimulation through our taste, smell, and perception neurochemical systems. This is a survival instinct. We desire and seek water with a thirst reflex, and food with a hunger reflex. We desire stimulation from human relationships and sex to continue our species' existence. Literally, the more stimulation, the better our nervous systems like it, even to the point of unhealthy excess.

The more concentrated artificial "food-like" substances we consume, the more they stimulate our neurochemistry and lead to weight gain. It is a destructive, vicious cycle. Unfortunately, in the modern commercial world, we fall prey to these primitive survival systems, which are exploited by unscrupulous marketing and the gratuitous manufacture and sale of unhealthy products.

The empowering news Is that you can make healthy lifestyle choices every day by using your grey thinking matter over the reactive white matter of your brain. You can decide what adequate stimulation is and avoid inappropriate or excessive stimulation.

Our bodies and society are about power and stimulation. An early psychologist named Dr Alfred Adler (1870-1937) theorized that Dr. Sigmund Freud (1856-1939) was wrong in his theory that all mental health issues were somehow tied to the desire for sex. Dr. Freud was right that both men and women had a deep passion for sex, but, in my opinion, it isn't the deepest driver of human behavior. Dr. Adler advocated that power was a more critical basic driver: power over your life circumstances, desires, and the actions of other humans.

I believe that the basic instinct and drive to survive, which commands us this very moment to seek stimulation, drives both power and sex. Unfortunately, when the drive is further stimulated to consume that which is destructive to our body, we not only lose power and our ability to have sex, but it can also take our lives.

Chapter Six
Why Do We Eat?

"The physician must be a student of humanity."
–Andrew Taylor Still, DO

History, our humanity, and science tell us we eat and drink to stay alive, ostensibly to reproduce the species. But, is that the only reason that we eat and drink? Hell, no!

We have many excuses for when to eat. Being both culturally and religiously Jewish, I relate to the experience of eating in many ways: It's a holiday, let's eat. It's not a holiday, let's eat. It's the Sabbath, let's eat. It's not the Sabbath, let's eat. We're celebrating something, let's eat. We're not celebrating something, let's eat. We're happy, let's eat. We're sad, let's eat. We're together, let's eat. We're lonely, let's eat. We're anxious, let's eat. We're depressed, let's eat. Eating is an expression of love and care. Oh hell, let's just EAT! There's always a "reason" to eat.

One can find numerous reasons to eat, beyond mere survival. We use eating as part of our rituals, culture, and for the neurostimulation it provides (which we'll discuss again soon). And of course, we eat for survival.

As essential as eating is, there are concerns and cautions associated with it. Understanding what triggers and motivates you is crucial to good health, as it informs decisions about what to eat and when to eat it.

People eat for a variety of reasons, not just hunger. People eat because they feel sad or happy. People eat when they meet with another person. People eat when they are lonely. People eat to gain weight. People eat to lose weight. The worst excuse of all is that people eat out of BOREDOM. People find seemingly endless reasons (excuses) to eat. But why?

Pattern of food intake

Have you ever noticed (shades of the late Andy Rooney of CBS' "60 Minutes" in the 1970s-1980s) the pattern in the way we consume food? From the first bite, each consecutive bite tends to be larger. Why? It is related to my hypothesis about an individual's innate programming, the concentration/stimulation theory.

We agree that humans enjoy being stimulated in a variety of ways; we see it as "pleasurable." Why? The concentration, duration, and frequency of the stimulus are the differences. For example, concentrated food derivatives, i.e., #notfood like ice cream, strongly and more acutely stimulates the brain's neurochemistry than food like lettuce. Our brains and bodies quickly habituate (that is, get used to) the quick, more powerful stimuli. Each subsequent bite must be either more concentrated or larger to generate the same pleasure response from our brain as the previous bite. This is precisely the reason that we take progressively larger bites as we eat. This is even more true when we consume concentrated food derivatives, or #notfood. The brain, nervous system, and other body organs constantly up-regulate and down-regulate receptors, given the concentration, intensity, and time of stimulation. That is habituation, or in laymen's terms, getting used to something. The same experience applies to all stimulatory and addictive substances, including sugar, cocaine, heroin, tobacco smoke, etc.

Each dose of a "drug" must grow stronger by being more concentrated and/or by taking a larger dose in a more rapid pattern or longer time of exposure, to elicit the same pleasure response as the first one. Doesn't this sound like everything you've ever heard about opiates like Percocet™ and heroin, for instance? This is why all the developed nations quickly became addicted to the trappings of their successes; so-called "luxury food" (kudos to Glenn Tilbrook of Squeeze, "I'll buy you an ice cream as big as your head;" his father's skiffle song). These "luxury" foods (#notfood) are loaded with sugar, saturated fat, cholesterol, and salt. "Food" created by the industrial food industry is #notfood—notice also that #notfood is also more concentrated than #realfood. A simple example of this is how Doritos™ chips compare to an ear of corn.

Over the last 100 years, most of the developed Western world has consumed luxury food as a primary food. These consumers have shunned genuine staple foods, like raw vegetables. The reality is that people around the globe crave the intense stimulation that #notfood brings, and the "food" industry knows it quite well.

The food industry's scientific research ignores the healthiest combinations of foods. Big food conglomerates ("Big Food") fund research that produces intense stimulation; these contain salt, fat, sugar, cholesterol, and other taste sensations. Note: In the 1980s, following court suits and government monetary penalties for years of deceptive practices, big tobacco companies acquired most of the major food companies. Ah, so now it makes more sense. Big Tobacco used their dependence and addiction research, and deceptive practices for the big food products they now own and sell. Consumers prefer these sensate substances driven by stimulation, rather than maintaining their best health. Human sensations related to food encompass smell, taste, mouthfeel, and sensory experience. Instead of using our "noggins" to think, plan, execute, and achieve a healthy diet, our body loses good health. My late father used to say, "Use your head for something other than a hat rack."

Food addiction

Plainly said, obesity is related to addiction. YES! Now you

know how and why. Some would say, "it's not your fault." But I say, "it may not be your fault, per se, but it is your problem. Fix it."

In psychology, psychiatry, and addiction medicine, there is a concept called "dual diagnosis." Most addicts, whether to #notfood or other drugs, have dual diagnoses. Each addicted person usually has not only a physical addiction but a clinical psychological or psychiatric diagnosis that is directly related, and one facilitates the other. Some people are clinically depressed and constantly try to fill the emotional and mental void with fattening #notfood. Others, with #notfood addiction, gain weight and become clinically depressed. This is the cycle of obesity and poor health that turns round and round. This is a quintessential example of the chicken-and-egg phenomenon. We don't know necessarily which came first, but we do know both are present, and they facilitate the existence of the other.

If a patient has experienced addiction or a dependence state, or knows someone who has, this "dual diagnosis" becomes clearer. If a person admits to an addiction, sees that it causes negative consequences, and shares a desire to fix it, he or she can make headway toward a cure, or at least learn to cope with it more healthily. However, when there is a dual diagnosis, a person cannot treat or end the addiction in any long-term sense. This person must confront and treat the mental health issue that caused them to be susceptible to the addiction. These are the so-called historical "demons" that one is subject to.

How many psychologists does it take to change a light bulb? It only takes one, but first, the light bulb must want to change.

Consider this dual diagnosis in the following way. You have a dinner table that has a problem. It bumps up and down during dinner, annoying the diners. If you have a four-legged table with one leg that is an inch shorter than the others, it is unstable. To compensate for instability, you can place magazines, books, or other items under the short leg, which may help. The props are required to minimize the bumping problem. The only way to fix the problem long-term, however, is to recognize that the short leg is causing the problem, and either lengthen it or replace it with a proper-length leg. Finding and addressing the stability problem makes the bumping problem solvable. Shoving things under the short table leg for a temporary fix never completely solves the problem.

Medical and psychological care are required to treat both diagnoses, mental and physical. Improving either is helpful but improving both will eventually lead to a more positive resolution to both problems. Concerning what we eat, eating healthy food and drinking water treats and ultimately prevents anxiety and depression, and deals with addiction, to an extent. Failure to do so means the poisons and addictive quality of the #notfood ingestion will resist and worsen the mental illness, thus complicating the task.

Consider "holism." It involves viewing and treating the body as an integrated unit consisting of many organ systems and cells. Recognizing this idea when considering healthy practices for our body harkens back to the late Andrew Taylor Still, DO, Asian Indian Yoga, Chinese medicine, and the early origins of health, disease, and body/mind treatments.

Dieting "one-mealers" fail

Some "on the go" individuals start their day with an acidic caffeine beverage (coffee or tea), with added sugar and saturated fat, and then go all day without eating or drinking adequate water until dinner. Does this sound familiar at all? Their dinner is large, and the accompanying beverage may be soda, wine, beer, coffee, or tea; still, no plain water. I call these people "one-mealers" or "feast/faminers." Their bodies enter starvation/famine mode and begin to use sugar stores, reabsorb fat, and muscle to meet their fuel needs. Their brain and kidneys initially release water into urine due to the diuretic effect of caffeine. Hours later, the body realizes that it is even further dehydrated and enters water conservation mode. At the end of the workday, they eat the last meal of their day (and may seek snacks later via the "reconsideration habit " to be discussed later). Their dinner is thought to provide a whole day's food, calories, or more, all at once. Soon after dinner and their late evening snacks, they go to bed.

Going to sleep with a full stomach is never a good idea for many reasons. A distended or full stomach can be physically uncomfortable when trying to sleep. The GI tract goes into action frantically to process the day's food all at once. The body goes into overdrive/feast mode. The extra calories stimulate the body to convert the excess energy into body fat. This intensifies during sleep. All this, and not to mention the gastroesophageal reflux of acid and partially digested food stewing all night long.

Those who eat large, highly caloric late-day/evening meals, especially when topped off with late-night snacks, tend to gain weight while they sleep. The "feast/faminers" have a high rate of obesity. They can't seem to understand why; they "only eat one meal a day." How could that be? Now you know why.

This is a rule about eating that we should all learn and practice: Food should be consumed in four to six small grazing meals, which are easier for the body to process. It also prevents the stomach from over-dissension or stretching out. Eventually, the stomach can lose its elasticity and stay in a larger form. This also damages stretch receptors that tell the brain that the stomach is filled. Imagine filling your car with gasoline and the pump had no pressure sensor, so you couldn't see the tank fill. Eventually, you would overfill the tank, wasting gasoline and damaging the car's paint finish, and the ground would become temporarily toxic. Don't overfill your tank of your stomach.

A second general rule about eating: We should eat healthy foods and avoid unhealthy foods altogether, #notfood.

A third rule is do not eat within 3-4 hours of going to bed. And, no late-night snacks, for sure.

Chapter Seven
Toxins

"The body's natural state is one of health and vitality."
– Andrew Taylor Still, DO

Toxins or poisons are any substance that, when put into or on the body, causes an undesirable reaction that can impair or destroy health.

Cyanide is a toxin. When ingested, cyanide poisons the processes that our bodies use to produce life-sustaining energy. When energy processes are interrupted for a prolonged period, cells die, organs die, and eventually the body dies.

Small amounts of toxins exert stress on the body's metabolism, immune, and repair systems, causing them to work too hard. In return, slivers of an organ may die, leaving fewer living organs to perform the same job; that's a lot of stress!

When a person drinks large amounts of alcohol at once or drinks alcohol intermittently over a long period, it attacks and kills cells in otherwise healthy living organs. The liver detoxifies ethanol (alcohol), but when the liver is overwhelmed by excessive ethanol over time, it can damage and/or destroy the liver and other organs, like the stomach and pancreas. The liver works to chemically change or detoxify ethanol so that it can be quickly eliminated from the body in a less harmful form.

Dr. Still predicted back in the early 1900s that by the end

of the Twentieth Century (1999), we in the U.S. would be a nation of overweight drug addicts (1990 Osteopathic Principles and Practices lecture, NYCOM/NYIT, New York College of Osteopathic Medicine). We know that two out of three people in the U.S. are overweight or obese. Besides obesity, too many people continue to smoke cigarettes, drink alcohol, smoke cannabis, make poor food choices, and take damaging over-the-counter drugs while consuming other selective toxins. How far was Dr. Still from the truth?

Cigarette smoking is one of the most significant sources of toxins in the world. Whether burned or chewed, tobacco products force the body to deal with many toxins. These include tar, nicotine, cyanide, benzene, toluene, carbon monoxide, and other combustion products.

Over time, as you may know, tobacco use directly causes many kinds of cancer, including lung, esophagus, tongue, and gum cancer. Indirectly, tobacco use causes breast, uterine, prostate, and skin cancer; that is, cancer of most, if not all, body organ systems. So what? Cancer, cancer, cancer. Who's afraid of the big, bad cancer?

The top two causes of death in 2025 in the United States are 1) heart disease, and 2) various forms of cancer. Smoking tobacco products can be a cause of both deadly conditions. It also plays a devastating part in many other disease states and destroys health.

Cigarette smoke has more than 4,000 poisons and toxins. The following is a partial list (in alphabetical order):

Acetone - paint stripper/nail polish remover

Acrolein - tear gas from World War I

Arsenic - rat poison

Butane - lighter fluid

Cadmium - a heavy metal from rechargeable batteries

Carbon monoxide - poison gas from car exhaust

Cyanide - rat poison

DDT – pesticide, tobacco plants may be treated with this

Formaldehyde - a preservative for dead bodies

Lead - toxin from old paint

Malathion – pesticide, tobacco plants may be treated with this

Methanol - jet fuel

Naphthalene - active ingredient in mothballs

Nicotine - an addictive stimulant

Parathion – pesticide, tobacco plants may be treated with this

Phenols - caustic compounds

Polonium - a radioactive element

Polynuclear aromatic hydrocarbons - cancer-causing

Tar - parking lot blacktop

Tar is composed of substances including benzene, toluene, naphthalene, anthracene, xylene, pyridine, ammonia, and phenols.

Tobacco products also cause chronic obstructive pulmonary disease (better known as emphysema), strokes, heart attacks, cancer, high blood pressure, and many other maladies.

Tobacco products "complicate" pregnancy. What does that mean, you ask? It can cause your unborn child to have asthma, low birth weight, respiratory distress syndrome, attention deficit/hyperactivity disorder, and other conditions that may lead to miscarriage and death of the fetus/preborn baby.

Why, in the most developed and "chemically safe" country in the world, does the U.S. government permit the sale of such deadly toxins for human consumption? This answer is, as you may have already guessed, MONEY! The biggest issue by far is that states and the federal government collect taxes on the production and sale of tobacco. Follow the money. Sound familiar to alcohol and cannabis (in some states)? Big Tobacco employs advertising agencies, lawyers, and market analysts to make the product appear appealing and to ensure its legality. This is done by expending vast amounts of money to convince each of us that not only are these products safe for others, but we, too, ought to use them.

Take, for example, the cigarette filter scam of the 1940s. Tobacco companies spent heavily to convince Americans that a filter made of cotton and paper created a "safer" cigarette. It did not, and the industry knew it. It was the biggest public health scam of its time. Later, the industry created "low tar" filters with ventilation holes to allegedly improve safety; however, these only required smokers to inhale harder to draw in the same amount of toxins. Again, another deadly farce.

People often justify their bad habits with anecdotes, like, "My great-grandmother lived to 77 years old and smoked three packs of cigarettes a day." Smokers try to excuse their tobacco use by pointing to people like her. In my practice, I've heard it all. The apocryphal great-grandmother story was a single, unique person, representing only herself, if she even existed at all. Perhaps she had a greater functional reserve or spare tissue to withstand the pollution and toxins. Living 77 years in her era was an exception but imagine how much healthier and longer she might have lived if she had had a healthy lifestyle. Without a doubt, she would have enjoyed a better quality of life, better mobility, and more clarity of thought.

My mother lived 67 years, after smoking two packs of "Salem Lights" a day, for about 51 of those years. She started smoking after school in Philadelphia in the 1950s. it was "adult," and even glamorous to smoke, when the tobacco industry gave so much money to the entertainment media for product placement; radio, TV, movies, etc. FYI, my mom died of a second type of cancer at 67 years old, in poor health.

Coffee (seeds of the Coffea plant, also called coffee cherries) and tea (Camellia sinensis leaf) also contain stimulants and toxins. The most notable is caffeine. It ultimately releases epinephrine and dopamine neurotransmitters, while blocking adenosine receptors that regulate relaxation/sleep in the body. It may make a person feel more awake, but it also increases their blood pressure and constricts their blood vessels. Some forms of tea, such as green tea, contain beneficial antioxidant constituents, but it's best to avoid the caffeinated variety. Rooibos, also known as "red tea," from South Africa, is a distinct plant that does not contain caffeine and is less acidic.

Caffeine results in a sense of "stress" or "fight or flight." Many people use the caffeine stimulation effect to become more alert and perform more strenuous physical work. As time passes and use continues, the body acclimates and habituates to the stimulation. This makes the same amount seem less stimulating. More concentration/stimulation evidence here.

Body systems compensate to reduce the effects of the stimulation over time. This is why people, line up at coffee shops and mini markets at dawn, must take in more caffeine to get the same effect, like cocaine. Caffeine is legal, and though no government taxes it directly, they may tax the products in which it is a key ingredient. Cocaine is illegal, and the government is trying to put the supply chain out of business while ignoring the damage that too much caffeine can do. Governments either tax a toxic substance or try to put it out of business by force. Both strategies have their risks and benefits, and thus, proponents and detractors.

The body habituates to toxic stimulants, and the "dosage" must continue to increase over time. This produces a new "normal" state of the push and pull between stress hormones and neurotransmitters, reducing the stimulatory effect. When a toxic stimulant is withdrawn, the body's blood vessels quickly dilate, causing withdrawal symptoms of headache and fatigue. This painful effect, usually a headache, literally and figuratively, causes a person to reduce discomfort and return to the stimulated state by making or buying another cup of coffee—they see it as a medical treatment, ironically. "*Sic transit gloria mondae*," which is Latin for glory is fleeting! This is why: to quit consuming these stimulant toxins, we must slowly taper down their intake over time to re-achieve balance and health.

What is the ultimate best answer about consuming toxins? Best advice: Avoid them all, including cigarettes, cigars, chewing tobacco, snuff, vaping, alcohol, caffeinated beverages (such as coffee, tea, and cola), processed sugars, and overtly saturated animal fats and cholesterol. After all, it's quite simple.

Chapter Eight
Water

"The normal flow of fluids is essential for the body's optimal function."
–Andrew Taylor Still, DO

Worried parents brought their pleasant and smart 12-year-old girl to the local hospital ER (Hospital Emergency room/department) for severe back pain one Sunday afternoon. Her mom, who raised several children and ran a retail business, and her dad, who practiced law, are both well-educated. They are nice, caring parents who want the best for their children.

The ER staff doctor explained to the parents that the medical workup showed nothing serious except for a trace of blood in her urine. This led the ER physician to order a kidney ultrasound imaging study. The study confirmed the presence of kidney stones.

Kidney stones produce one of the most painful conditions a person can experience while the stone passes down the ureters from the kidneys to the bladder and finally out the urethra. The diagnosis and the pain that this young girl would suffer disturbed the doctor; it disturbed her parents and the girl more. The doctor shook his head in amazement that a young, healthy, educated 12-year-old girl could have such a painful problem.

Her family had no known history of metabolic problems that could cause these stones in relatives. The most likely cause was chronic dehydration for years. In my opinion, most often, kidney stones, gall bladder stones, and similar conditions can be prevented with daily hydration throughout life. Many doctors do not even ask about or give suggestions about a patient's lifestyle choices. I, and precious few others, do,

A lack of sufficient, regular daily water intake leads to concentration of compounds in the kidneys that form stones, most frequently the calcium oxalate type. These kidney stones cause pain while stationary, from urine backup swelling up the kidney(s), and excruciating pain when passing down the urinary tract. They were likely preventable by increased healthy daily water intake.

Water for a healthy life

Water is the most crucial element in our survival and for maintaining our health. Most people in the USA are dehydrated daily. First, people in third- and second-world countries may not have access to clean (potable) drinking water. The same can perhaps be said for some urban centers in first-world countries. Secondly, some individuals do not care to urinate more than twice a day (the laziness factor). Third, people do not make drinking water a priority in their daily activities; worse still, they often give it no thought.

The average human body consists of more than 27 trillion cells. Single cells were first observed by the Dutch researcher Antonie van Leeuwenhoek (1632-1723), the "Father of Microbiology, during the 1670s. He designed and used the first primitive microscope to study simple items beginning with cork. He described those cells as "little rooms" in the cork structure.

Today, we understand that cells are the fundamental units that make up our design and structure. Cells are also used to describe bacteria (perhaps we are distantly related?).

Why, then, is water so important? This story begins on a most basic level: the cell. To perform their function correctly, cells always rely on a fresh supply of clean water. Cells cannot adequately perform their function without a certain amount of water, i.e., converting energy, building new cells, and carrying out the specific tasks of each organism in the body. In my experience, it's not the infection or disease process that drives you to the ER of a hospital, but the dehydration that it can cause or accompany it.

Each cell is suspended in a slight saltwater bath (normal saline, for example). Water brings nutrients to the cell; it assists in transporting away impurities and waste products. Thus, a constant flow of water is critical to the cell's survival, the organ's survival, and to the health and survival of each human body.

Our body is composed primarily of water. Water makes up our blood, lymph, and cerebrospinal fluid and makes everything move. It enables us to use our senses: see, smell, hear, feel, taste. Before birth, we live and breathe in amniotic fluid water for nine months. We come from water and therefore need a constant water intake to live and function.

The body constantly uses and loses water as it carries out its metabolic processes. We lose water (and salt) through sweat, breath, urine, and feces, among other means. The body's water supply must be constantly replenished. We can survive for up to a month without food, but we will die in only 7 days without water.

We get water through the liquids we drink and the food we eat. Vegetables and fruits, for example, have a high-water content. Eating vegetables and fruits daily is vital not only to nutrition but also to hydration.

Beverages with a large amount of added sugar, such as sodas and colas, contain so much sugar that they have little relative water. Caffeine in beverages, such as coffee, tea, and cola, acts as a diuretic, causing the body to eliminate water through urine. Alcoholic beverages, too, are diuretics. These add to dehydration (not enough water). I can't reinforce this enough.

Drinks and beverages are not mainly water but have many dissolved particles and active substances that can deplete your body of water instead of hydrating it.

The gastrointestinal (GI) tract acts like a typical sewage processing plant, or perhaps vice versa. Proper food processing requires adequate water intake and thorough chewing of food. Swallowing sends the food and water into the digestive system for processing. The mouth adds mild acids and digestive enzymes to the stomach acid with its strong acids, pH 1-2, and more digestive enzymes. The stomach churns this mixture, called chyme. Water is necessary so the mix can move along, and elements can be absorbed through the wall of the small intestine. The large intestine (bowel) then reabsorbs the water back out of the chyme for "recycling," returning it to the system. The rectum is the final stop for this, now firm, more solid waste feces ("poop"), which is expelled from the body through defecation, ideally on cue.

Water also transports blood elements and cellular fluids to and out of the GI tract. The kidneys filter the water and eliminate cellular waste in the form of urine, which is stored in the bladder for removal through urination. Urine output is a reliable indicator of hydration, dehydration, and water status when balanced against water intake.

Most people should aim to consume four to six glasses of clean water daily (approximately 1.5 gallons, or 5.7 liters total) as part of their daily diet. This must be a priority. Considering that caffeine and alcohol are diuretics that signal the kidneys to excrete water from the body, it becomes more crucial to either reduce or eliminate caffeine and alcohol intake. Yes, you will urinate, or go to the bathroom, 4-6 times per day, but this is really healthy and normal. This enables us to maximize our health.

It has been said many times in many ways: "One solution to pollution is dilution." This I learned at the environmental college where I earned a BS degree in Food Science Research. The greater amount of fresh water you take into your body, the less that ecological or other pollutants negatively affect you.

We have explored why we all need adequate and ample water. Then, why is the average person dehydrated?

Our bodies consist of over 60% water. Isn't it amazing that a bag of water, like us, can do so much harm to ourselves, others, and the environment? We are bags of water with particles, i.e., various elements and minerals floating about inside us.

Good health is achieved and maintained by a constant intake of water. A. T. Still, DO, the founder of Osteopathic medicine, wrote about this in the late 1800s. Ironically, this fact has been known for so long, but far too few people have written about it since. A pragmatic observation reveals that adequate water intake apparently doesn't fit our modern technological lifestyle since the Industrial Revolution.

We lose water in various ways on a routine basis. It is lost through both sensible and insensible losses, including chemical reactions in the body, sweating, urine, feces, and exhaling moist air, among others. The body is a great compensator. It can function to some extent on moderate amounts of water that it derives from liquids and foods. But, to really be at the pinnacle of health, one requires 32 to 64 ounces of water per day, in addition to the water content of foodstuffs.

There is an excellent (TV and Web advertising) beverage myth: "Soft drinks quench thirst." When I was in my early teens, I played baseball and football with the other children in the neighborhood. After a summer day of active playing, I would come home thirsty. I could drink a two-liter (half gallon at the time) bottle of cola/soda (or pop, depending on where you're reading this) and still be thirsty. How could this be? Shouldn't it have quenched my thirst? The answer is no!

Most soft drinks are loaded with high-fructose corn syrup, sucrose, dextrose, and other sugar sweeteners. They all translate into concentrated forms of sugar. These sugars make the products sweet, appealing to the market audience the drink is targeting. Far too many individuals develop a dependence on these beverages and wrongly believe they fill the need for daily water intake.

Not only are sodas a source of overwhelming calories, but they are also a source of other detrimental particles. Surely, one can see that we do not need harmful particles floating about in our bag of water, gumming up the mix.

We require a specific balance of free water and particles to function correctly. Each cell uses its energy to balance the mix of particles and water inside its borders. Cells and the overall human body have an easier time dealing with (relatively) too much water than (relatively) too many particles. We need more just plain water in our daily diets.

Please note that increasing your daily water intake may result in slightly more frequent urination. This is a good sign, not (just) an annoying inconvenience. It reminds us that we are doing the right thing and keeping our cells happy and healthy, not to mention our kidneys! Remember, "One solution to pollution is dilution." It lessens the disturbance to your body systems or reduces the impact. The same can be said about the environment.

Chapter Nine
Food

"Let food be thy medicine and medicine be thy food."
– Hippocrates of Kos (460-370 BC)

Don't panic! This is not a harangue about changes you must make or fail outright, which would seem hopeless and utterly resistant to any change. Instead, it presents a healthy view of what can be. Diet has become an epithet, or proverbial "four-letter bad word," over the last few decades, although it remains four letters. Merriam-Webster defines "diet" as "Food and drink regularly provided or consumed." Everyone who eats regularly has a diet. It is not an epithet, but only a catch-all word for the staple and way in which you eat regularly.

"To diet" is the hated phrase of intention. It means, "To restrict oneself to small amounts or special kinds of food in order to lose weight," says Merriam-Webster. Ah, there's the misery we have all grown accustomed to.

If you live, and wish to continue to do so, you will be "on a diet," for better or worse, your whole life. You can be purposeful in your eating style or eat haphazardly at the mercy of whatever is put before you. We are going to the better part of that cliché.

Health is the goal of a lifestyle plan, built on simple rules or guidelines. This section outlines some basic tools for food selection. It is not about calorie counting, weighing portions, or complex equations to apply.

Some diet plans are so complicated that trying to figure them out leaves you little or no time to eat. There is truth in "A calorie is a calorie," as the saying goes. Any diet plan that restricts calories below daily caloric energy usage will result in weight loss. Although diets that restrict caloric intake will help you lose weight, they are not always healthy over the long term. Calorie-counting diets work in the short term, but they fail if you don't limit yourself to the minuscule portions, especially of the same concentrated high-calorie foods that made you fat in the first place. The problem arises when you complete the likely expensive fad-diet program, and you are still unsure how to purchase and prepare healthy food for life.

Other weight-loss plans have you eating from plastic bags of prepared food. This is portion control. Unless you are a paying customer (member), it is nearly impossible to see the ingredients before purchasing the food. Also, these plans keep you dependent on the program for the foreseeable future, with no end in sight. Again, here you are, eating the concentrated, low-water, high-calorie foods that made you unwell in the first place.

There are many diet plans available, ranging from omnivorous (all are on the menu), carnivorous (animal-based), herbivorous (vegetarian), regional diets (such as Mediterranean or Japanese), and fad diets, including Atkins (pre-paleo), fasting, option-limited diets (the pineapple diet, which came and went) and option-emphasized diets (most common fad diets). Only relatively recently has "diet" been taken to mean loathsome, restrictive eating plans.

Most "diets, or diet plans," are so narrow and restrictive that you can't stick to them for very long. The common experience is that individuals lose serious weight, feel good about themselves, and then return to old habits and their former sloppy weight. Each time a person finds themselves staring at their once-again enlarged belly, it evokes a sense of hopelessness, which often leads to increased consumption and undesirable results; food as comfort. Doesn't that sound like what happens in drug abuse and dependence?

Health Is Number One Lifestyle (HINO)

Any diet or plan that significantly reduces calorie intake through food choices will lead to weight loss. Again, "a calorie is a calorie." Calories are the measurement of the potential energy contained in a food or substance when acted upon by the body during digestion and absorption. Proteins and carbohydrates provide 4 calories per gram, while fats provide 9 calories per gram. Fats are therefore more calorie dense. Calories, though important, are only part of the story of achieving and maintaining best health.

The raw vegan vegetarian diet may be optimal for most in the ideal world, but it faces many challenges. The real-world circumstances of daily life can interfere. Vegan and vegetarian diets require planning and effort to obtain fresh foods and store them properly, either immediately or briefly in the refrigerator. Most plant proteins, individually, do not provide all the essential amino acids necessary for human life. These must be complemented with others to ensure complete, crucial amino acids for life. Hint: Except for what plant?

The acronym from the Food Science college curriculum, freshman Introduction to Nutrition class, was Private Tim Hall, or PVT TIM HaLL. Phenylalanine, Valine, Threonine, Tryptophan, Isoleucine, Methionine, Histidine, Leucine, Lysine.

Actually, soybeans supply complete amino acid protein. Soy is flexible and can be prepared in many ways. I call it "nature's near-perfect food," due to its plant-based, protein, nutrient, and water content.

The Mediterranean diet, as is typical in Italy and Greece, is a healthy option. It includes some fish, animal meat, eggs, and cheese, rather than just vegetables, fruit, and grains, which are typically found in a vegan diet. Mediterranean people tend to be physically active, drink more water, and eat more fresh, unprocessed foods. Anyone who travels to Italy will tell you, anecdotally, that the food tastes so much better there. The portions were likely smaller abroad than those found in the U.S., with a lower calorie load and density per meal.

This brings us to the Health Is Number One (HINO) lifestyle nutrition plan. The HINO diet combines the healthiest aspects of the vegan and vegetarian diets with some of the most satisfying features of the Mediterranean diet. It all starts with a diet primarily of vegetables, excluding only starchy tubers like potatoes and sweet potatoes. Add fish (not shellfish, due to cholesterol and toxin content) and egg whites (not the yolks due to saturated fats and cholesterol) for protein, and a bit of whole grains and fruits. Eat nuts, legumes/beans, and seeds. It is that simple!

HINO staple food class is vegetables for their high nutrient density, low calorie nature, relatively low particle concentration, and water content. Add soy, fish, and egg white for protein, along with whole grains and fruit for fiber and energy. HINO is pesce (fish), ovo (egg white) vegetarian in structure. It is simple, satisfying, fulfilling, and beneficial to one's health. It is both satisfying and a best health winner, in my opinion.

Sugars, Starches, and Carbohydrates

Sugars are a type of dietary carbohydrate. There are simple sugars, complex sugars, and starches that turn into sugar in the body. Fiber-containing food generally includes digestible sugars and starches in the same food (i.e., cereal grains, oatmeal, and granola). It is advantageous to eat whole grains (carbohydrates, i.e., sugars, starches, with fiber) in the morning as they require the gut to work harder to fully digest the mix. If you eat them at dinner, they are likely to remain in your stomach all night, leading to acid reflux, indigestion, and weight gain. You may also wake up in the morning with a bloated, gassy abdomen; not much of a fun feeling. I understand that avoiding grains is the basis for the "Grain Belly" book and diet program by William Davis, MD. Some of my colleagues, like Lynn Flynn, MD, and Richard Urso, MD, and John Littell, MD who champion animal product emphasis diets, will say the same.

The mainstream media constantly talks about sugar. Many diet plans reduce or eliminate sugars. Sugars are a natural constituent of real food and provide energy; however, a few words of explanation would help clarify our understanding of the matter.

The public and media think of sugar to mean only one thing: sucrose or dextrose or "table sugar." Sugar, as a class, also includes glucose, galactose, fructose, lactose, and other naturally occurring energy-supplying molecules. The food industry concentrated sugars as sucrose; it is #notfood as our bodies and ecosystem intended. Food manufacturers isolated sucrose by hyper-concentrating sugar molecules from sugar cane or sugar beets into white crystals. Sucrose is added to beverages and food products. Our brains love the stimulation of hyper-concentrated sugar, and we buy it uncontrollably from our supermarkets, stores, and so-called fast-food restaurants. Nature does not make sucrose "table sugar," the food industry does.

The food industry has also figured out how to make high-fructose corn syrup. The Corn Refiners Association estimates that more than 40,000+ packaged foods in the U.S. contain high-fructose corn syrup. The food industry knows that our "sweet tooth" drives us to buy products, so they concentrate artificial sugars in our food and beverage products. Fructose is cheaper to make and obtain than sucrose. That is why the food industry at large uses it preferentially. It is ultra-sweet, easy to add to food products, shelf-stable, and as passionately addictive as sucrose. Oh, I should add that it is so cheap, at least in part, due to the U.S. government subsidizing corn farming and production. So, the government has been using tax dollars (read that, your money!) to pay for factory farms and corn processors to help big food/tobacco companies to profit from keeping you addicted, unhealthy, and fat. Imagine that.

Beverage plants load up soda, pop, cola, ginger ale, root beer (soft drinks) with artificially concentrated sugars like sucrose and/or high-fructose corn syrup. The industry knows that our public buys them and consumes them with reckless abandon, to the point (and beyond) of diseases like obesity, diabetes, cancer, heart attack, and stroke. Incredibly, the U.S. government subsidizes large corn product agribusiness companies that grow and refine corn into corn syrup, which is then used to produce high-fructose corn syrup. There is always a ready supply awaiting your palate, everywhere from the supermarket to your pantry.

Let us learn to avoid sucrose (table sugar) and high-fructose corn syrup like the plague it is. They are #notfood and when consumed, they cause disease and obesity.

Keep an Eye on Blood Sugar

Each of us should undergo an annual blood sugar screening at your annual health maintenance assessment, or HMA, as I call it. It can be conducted by your trusted family physician in two basic forms: fasting blood sugar and HbA1c, or simply A1c, as is commonly known. Fasting blood sugar measurement at a lab requires a 12-hour overnight fast to standardize the results. Some use an 8-hour fast, but I've found, over 25+ years of osteopathic family medical practice, that often, food remains in the stomach all night. This, in turn, leads to factitious or erroneous fasting glucose results. Factitious refers to results that appear incorrect for the situation but are actually influenced by a confounding variable or circumstance. We use a dedicated 12-hour fast, from, say, 6 PM to 6 AM, for example. This reduces the timing variable confound. This number should ideally be less than 100. If the result is 100 or more, it indicates impaired fasting glucose, or prediabetes.

Although many of my peers and the American Diabetes Association (ADA) believe diabetes begins at a fasting blood glucose level of 125, I believe diabetes starts at 100. Long-term sugar, called HbA1c, should be less than 5.7%. Hemoglobin A1c measures the amount of sugar stuck to the outside of a red blood cell. Because a red blood cell lives for about 90 days in blood circulation, it provides a 90-day snapshot of a person's general blood sugar control. If this value is above 5.6%, it indicates impaired glucose tolerance. I believe that this is where diabetes begins, not at 6.5% which the ADA and U.S. federal government currently promulgates and promotes.

A 3-hour glucose tolerance test, with 100g of glucose syrup, should take place for those with blood relatives with a history of diabetes, who are overweight or obese, and those who have unexplained symptoms or otherwise cannot achieve their ideal weight. Most labs use 75g for men and non-pregnant women and 100g glucose load for pregnant women. This additional testing consists of a 12-hour fast and begins with the measurement of fasting blood glucose. Then the patient is asked to drink a concentrated sugar beverage with a 75g or 100g glucose load. Blood sugar is measured every half hour for three hours to watch the body's response to the induced high sugar load. The body should be able to maintain blood sugar levels below 140 for three hours and return them to a baseline of under 100. If the sugar level starts above 100, exceeds 140, or fails to return to less than 100 after three hours, the test result indicates impaired glucose tolerance. Prediabetes FBS >99, A1c >5/6%, oral glucose tolerance test >140, or at least 150, should be reclassified as diabetes. The numbers I use and recommend, as above, should be the values that define diabetes, from my perspective. Values above the normal range and indeed abnormal when unconfounded by factitious results. When numbers exceed the normal range, disease ensues. This is why we all should consider reclassifying impaired fasting glucose, impaired glucose tolerance, and prediabetes as diabetes.

Hypoglycemia to hyperglycemia

Our instructors in Osteopathic (D.O.) medical school taught us about hypoglycemia (low blood sugar) and diabetes/hyperglycemia (high blood sugar). We conceptualized that they were polar opposites and didn't occur in the same patients. We were taught that they were different diseases with other causes, symptoms, and outcomes. In practice, I have learned differently by observation and testing over decades of practice and thereby, taught by tens of thousands of patients.

The human body should eat as often as babies do, grazing every two to three hours, in my opinion. Instead, in the modern industrialized world, we are dogma-committed to three meals a day: breakfast, lunch, and dinner. In the reality of working life, many people usually have nothing but a cup of coffee (caffeinated acid) with cream (saturated bovine lactyl secretion fat) and concentrated crystalline concentrated sugar instead of breakfast. This, just after breaking their daily fast, is 12 hours of fasting. Another reason why breakfast is an important meal of the day. Lunch is often a sandwich made with salted animal meat and cheese (saturated fat and cholesterol) on white bread (starch), accompanied by deep-fried salted potato chips or French fries (dearly loved #notfood mess for most folks).

Sometime during the day, when a person senses a slowdown, he or she will grab something close, convenient, concentrated calorie-dense, such as a candy bar, a piece of cake, or a cookie, full of sugar and perhaps fat, and/or a caffeinated sugar soda. Their body is working hard to process these sugar- and saturated fat-laden foods. The sugars worsen the tired feeling with the body ramping up its digestion and self-defense mechanisms. This is why many people turn to caffeinated beverages to artificially boost their energy and get back to work.

Dinner is commonly an ideal family time, when we historically gather to indulge in animal meat and carbohydrates. Milk, sodas, or coffee are on the table. Perhaps a glass of wine. Water is not generally seen on the table.

Traditionally, dessert follows dinner, filling us with more sugar, starch, and fat. Soon after, we fall asleep, and our bodies scramble madly to process the concentrated extra calories, storing them as fat, which we gradually notice accumulating on our waistline or other undesirable areas of our body over time. "A moment on the lips, a lifetime on the hips," rings true.

Our bodies are not fans of this relatively new, concentrated-calorie food derivative diet and the high frequency of concentrated #notfood eating. Our ancestors used to graze multiple times a day, not binge frequently. When we skip a meal, whether on purpose (our "diet") or because we are too busy, our blood sugar drops (hypoglycemia). This can lead to fatigue and irritability, and we often grab the first food product that is nearby; usually #notfood snacks. When the concentrated sugar calories enter our bloodstream, the pancreas releases insulin rapidly to try to lower the blood sugar back to its previous level. The previous level, however, has been elevated to new, prolonged heights. We store these calories as fat.

Over time, given our poor eating habits (diet), we tend to gain weight. Our body has increased difficulty getting sugars under control, and we develop diabetes (hyperglycemia, obesity, and vascular blood vessel disease). It is a vicious cycle.

I see patients who are stuck in the middle of this cycle as they go from hypoglycemia to hyperglycemia at different points during the day. This is one of the factors that causes obesity and diabetes, now at epidemic levels in the developed industrial world. Now you can understand how slender people may experience symptomatic hypoglycemia and eat concentrated #notfood. Then the body stores the excess calories, over time, as fat.

As the body becomes obese, there is a predisposition for hyperglycemia. This, in turn, becomes obesity and diabetes, resulting in symptomatic hyperglycemia. In traditional medical teachings, we were taught polyphagia, polydipsia, and polyuria. These symptoms may also include fatigue, weight gain, thirst, urinary frequency, hunger, vision changes, and vascular disease.

We are creatures of habit. Most of us prefer the usual places, times, foods, drinks, and circumstances in our daily lives. In the developed world, we have the benefit of food security and the ready availability of water and food. But, the food/tobacco industry has co-opted our food system, with the help of your tax money and government programs, into #notfood security. For the politicians, it ensures industry campaign donations to buy advertising to get re-elected. For the food/tobacco industry, it ensures and insures big profits. For you, it ensures constant, concentrated, addictive temptation at every turn. Will you fall for it again and again?

We can and must prevent the cycle from starting, or break it if it has begun, by taking charge of our lifestyle. Again, hearing my father's voice, "Use your head as something other than a hat rack."

Stop drinking your fat on

Carbonated beverages have a fascinating history. Before the twentieth century, they were not found anywhere in the marketplace. People, besides their own fermented alcoholic beverage experiments, primarily drank water. They also drank natural, unpasteurized fruit cider, which was uncooked and unsterilized, leaving its nutrients intact if consumed shortly after it was produced.

Pharmacists at their local, independently owned shops searched for various drinks that could have potential medicinal applications. Dr. John Sith Pemberton is credited with inventing Coca-Cola in 1886. Before he died in the late 1890s, Pemberton sold his formula to Asa Candler, who incorporated the Coca-Cola Company in 1892.

Mixed with carbonated water, Jacobs' Pharmacy sold the

first "drinks" on May 8, 1886. The original formulation included cocaine(!), absurd and unacceptable by today's standards.

In 1914, the federal government made cocaine a controlled substance and banned it from Coca-Cola or any other similar beverage. In response, Coca-Cola reformulated the beverage, adding sugar (dextrose), "caramel coloring," caffeine, and other "natural" and "artificial" flavors, which were not disclosed on the label as they are proprietary to the company. The company substituted the stimulant drug caffeine as a legal replacement for cocaine.

Many other companies followed Coca-Cola's lead with products that include Pepsi, Royal Crown (RC), and other familiar brand names. Over the last 100 years, these ultra-sweet, ultra-concentrated, and ultra-stimulating artificial beverages have taken center stage at the American drink fountain. Many mixed alcohol drinks use these sodas as a primary base into which alcohol is added, which is turned into sugar in the body as well.

Each ingredient in these artificially formulated beverages poses a health hazard to the consumer. The sucrose "table sugar" commonly known as sugar, formally known as dextrose, is a potent calorie source that is much more concentrated than the natural sugar cane and sugar beets from which it is extracted and artificially concentrated. This causes two problems. The first is that sugar is already a concentrated source of calories. This contributes significantly to the obesity epidemic in the developed world. The body takes the calories in and must break them down to digest them. This causes the second problem.

The body needs water to dilute these artificially concentrated sugars. It must steal water from the circulatory blood and lymphatic systems. This creates artificial body fluid concentration elsewhere in the body. This, in turn, forces the kidneys to retain water, preventing it from passing out of the body in urine. A constant water intake is necessary to flush out water and toxins to maintain the concentration of body fluids at normal, low levels. When the concentration rises to high levels for extended periods, waste and toxins remain in the system longer, and commonly, calcium oxalate type gall bladder and kidney stones form.

The addition of caffeine worsens the concentration effect of these beverages. It tells the brain to signal the kidneys to release more water than usual, resulting in a diuresis or diuretic effect of urine.

Caffeine is a legal stimulant drug. To most people, caffeine is relatively harmless. After all, they find it readily available in beverages like sodas, coffee, and tea. They believe that caffeine is a safe additive to food. Although it can increase your ability to stay awake and do more muscular work, it does come at a risky price. Caffeine can also cause increased heart rate, high blood pressure, anxiety, and insomnia. With all these problems and no package insert or informed consent, caveat emptor: "let the buyer beware."

Let me be clear: Caffeine is simply not a safe drug for use or as an additive to food or beverages. It leads to dependence, addiction, and multiple disease states, including but not limited to hypertension, cardiac arrhythmias like atrial fibrillation, anxiety, sleep disturbances, and many other issues.

Side note: Interestingly, when middle-aged or older folks get a persistent run of atrial fibrillation, causing them health risks of blood clots, etc., cardiologists are reticent to inquire about a patient's use of caffeine at all. After all, who wants to tell an individual that their own habits may be responsible for their disease risk and symptom woes? That is, when you can avoid confrontation, prescribe expensive and toxic medications, and do expensive heart surgical procedures, like ablation? Trusted colleagues, are you listening?

It never ceases to amaze me when my patients who haven't embraced the reality of their lifestyle and habits, will begrudgingly take poisons, and have risky medical "procedures," so that they don't have to confront messes of their own constant making. Now is your chance to learn, change, and get it right!

In the early 2000s, researchers reported that "caramel coloring" added to soft drinks wasn't the food industry's heat-treated sugar "candy." Rather, caramel coloring is a complicated mix of chemicals that may cause cancer. Caramel coloring, like caffeine, is not a safe food additive and should not be consumed.

Carbonated water seemed safe, and the bubbles provide these beverages with a unique mouthfeel. The fundamental problem is that the human digestive tract does not "take kindly" to bubbles of carbon dioxide introduced into the human digestive tract. They are counterproductive to the GI tract's purpose, which is to move digested food smoothly. The gas that makes carbonated water "pleasurable" in mouthfeel, when ingested into the GI tract, causes distention of all the structures and blows them up like balloons. The Germans call it "magen blasse." If you have ever had a bad case of "gas," you now understand the result.

Charged with carbonated water, these beverages are a major unnecessary cause of gas and many other problems. Internally trapped gas causes pain, burping, hiccups, food and acid reflux, vomiting and, later in the digestive process, flatulence and explosive feces ("sorry about that, chief," in the immortal words of Don Adams as Maxwell Smart, Secret Agent 86 of Control from the 1960-1970s TV series Get Smart, by Mel Brooks and Buck Henry). CO2 may also exert pressure on the normal flora, including bacteria and yeast, that normally reside in our gastrointestinal tracts. These commensal organisms help us digest and process food, but when pressured, they may die or give way to pathogenic disease-causing microorganisms.

Chapter Ten
Fats, Oils, & Cholesterol

"Using the 5 Pillars or the 4 Lines of Evidence, there exists biochemistry, randomized trials, epidemiology and Centenarian data that indicate that diets lower in saturated fats (reduced or absent meats, cheeses, butter, pastries, lard, ghee) promote health and reduce the risk of heart disease. No single new study can upend 70 years of research even if a new study can get inordinate and inappropriate praise in the media. While nutritional science can be challenging, using the methods here will help you make healthy decisions about your diet, always favoring plant-based selections. Do not believe all media headlines. They can be bought or, at a minimum, influenced by a flow of dollars that generates clickbait headlines."

–Joel Kahn, MD, cardiologist

Start by minimizing saturated fats and cholesterol. These come from animal sources such as cheese, so-called "red meat," pork, ("the other white meat") so-called "white" meat poultry (fowl/birds like chicken and turkey), butter, animal fat, and deep-fried foods. Do not be fooled; oil is just another name for fat, but it is liquid at room temperature, so it is called oil. Saturated oils, such as those found in tallow/meat products, peanuts, coconuts, and other tropical oils, are particularly unhealthy. Less saturated oil, such as whole or extra virgin olive oil, is a better choice.

Fats, also known as lipids, play a crucial role in energy metabolism. However, most Americans never suffer from a fat deficiency. On the contrary, most Americans take in too much dietary animal fat each day.

Dietary fat is an essential component of a healthy daily diet. The healthiest fats are those from plant sources. These include avocadoes, soy and other beans/legumes, nuts, and seeds. They are not only healthy food, but they make convenient snacks.

Saturated fats are primarily found in animal products, such as "red" meat, pork, poultry, and dairy products like whole milk, and concentrated dairy products like cheese and butter. These products should only be minimally consumed; i.e., lesser amounts at a meal, or ideally, not consumed at all, in my opinion. Ice cream, butter, and cheese are highly concentrated food derivatives, #notfood. The are also inflammatory in nature for most people, another reason to avoid them.

Fats and oils are closely related. Fat differs from oil only because fat is solid at room temperature. Oil is a liquid at room temperature. Chemically, fats and oils have the same effect on your body, depending on their type and origin. Fish oil, however, is a healthy source of antioxidants, while saturated animal fat may increase cardiovascular risk and the risk of colon cancer.

Saturated fat is the most problematic of all. It can cause plaque to form, which is deposited in the walls of blood vessels. This can cause heart disease, strokes, hypertension, kidney failure, etc. Lard and beef tallow are among the worst fats to use. Nut-derived oils such as peanut and sesame, as well as coconut, are highly saturated. Trans fatty acids, which are created for use by the food industry, are also dangerous to healthy blood vessels.

Fast foods like cheeseburgers and French fries are high in saturated fat. They also have high cholesterol and salt content. These deep-fried carbohydrates (sugars and starches) are likely the worst of the worst for their disease-causing potential. Vegetables, nuts, beans, whole fibrous grains, and fruit are healthier choices, in that order, in my opinion.

Unsaturated fats and oils are better for your body. Unsaturated oils, such as olive oil, are considered healthy options. Cooking tip: Use whole olive oil to cook with as it has a higher smoke point. That means that it doesn't burn at lower temperatures, causing potentially toxic side-products. Use extra virgin olive oil for dressings and to top foods as desired. Extra virgin olive oil, or the first cold pressing output, has more anti-oxidants and nutrients, but a lower smoke point. It tends to burn when you cook with it at higher temperatures. Check the labels on food products at the store. Federal law requires that labels on processed food products show the type and amount of fat they contain.

Processed food manufacturers want you to buy their products. Therefore, they will do anything to make them taste better; this includes adding more fat, cholesterol, or sugar (sucrose or fructose, for example). Fat-free foods often contain added sugar for this reason. Fat-free = high sugar, sugar-free = high fat, fat and sugar-free = high salt. Be careful to select foods wisely.

Remember that eating less animal fat, in general, is better.

Another myth about fat is cholesterol. Fat is hard on your digestive system and can lead to a poor water-soluble nutrient absorption, in my opinion. Cholesterol and fat are chemically related but are not the same thing. For instance, a food may have no cholesterol but is high in fat, such as peanut butter. Aww, I can hear the groans and moans.

In the 1980s, when the government and big pharma moved toward exclusively blaming cholesterol for all cardiovascular diseases, the food industry responded. "Big Food," started labeling cholesterol, or the lack thereof, in food product packaging. Cholesterol comes only from animal sources. It is not found in plant sources.

Skippy ™ brand peanut butter, which was owned by Best Foods at that time, put on their label that it was "cholesterol free peanut butter." They implied that Skippy ™ was different from other peanut butters. The truth is that ALL peanut butters are cholesterol free! Because of this, the U.S. FDA made them change their labelling to reflect that the entire class of food was cholesterol free, not only by source, but by definition. Today you will notice that peanut butters are labeled, "peanut butter: a cholesterol free food," which more clearly communicates the truth.

Not all peanut butter is the same. Many contain salt, sugar, emulsifiers, preservatives, and more. I recommend the "natural" variety, but you must read the label always. "Ingredients: peanuts," should be the primary labeling.

Natural peanut butter, although it contains no cholesterol, is high in plant fat. This is because the peanut itself is where the peanut plant stores its energy in the form of fat. Natural peanut butter does contain high-quality protein and other essential nutrients. However, it is crucial to be mindful of overusing it due to its caloric density, owing to its fat content.

Currently, it is understood that saturated fat, trans fat, and cholesterol cause health problems. Be safe and sure. Minimize saturated fat, trans-fat, and cholesterol in your diet.

Fiber

To maintain good gastrointestinal health, it is essential to increase your dietary fiber intake. Most people in the United States consume far too little fiber. Fiber is a part of food that is resistant to digestion. It is found in grain products, fruits, and vegetables. The most common American diet is high in fat and cholesterol but low in fiber. This is one of the factors that has resulted in an extremely high incidence of heart and blood vessel disease in the United States.

So, what benefit do you receive from eating fiber in your diet? I'm glad that you asked.

A healthy diet must consist of adequate amounts of fiber and water. Fiber is the part of food that your gastrointestinal tract cannot digest. Dietary fiber is the sum of fiber in foods, and the level in grams that appears on nutritional food labels. Soluble fiber mixes with water. Insoluble fiber does not mix well with water. Fiber does not produce energy or give nutrients.

Insoluble fiber is terrific for your health. It adds bulk to your stool, making bowel movements less stressful. This reduces the risk of hemorrhoids and other problems. Insoluble fiber moves food through your system at a faster rate. Fiber helps move carcinogens and toxins along so that they are less likely to exert harmful effects. To strengthen your skeletal muscles, you lift weights at the gym. By bulking up your stools, insoluble fiber helps strengthen your intestinal muscles. Over many years, this will help prevent serious problems such as diverticulosis and diverticulitis.

Soluble fiber is a gummy substance that appears in vegetables, fruit, and a few processed foods. It reduces the amount of cholesterol absorbed in your small intestine. This can lower blood cholesterol levels. Additionally, the food scientist, or the well-trained cook for that matter, will add soluble fiber and gums to food to make fluids thicker or give a more satisfying feel in your mouth.

Fiber's Essential Purposes

Fiber serves two purposes: to make the intestine strong and to "clean house." The gastrointestinal (GI) tract extends from mouth, down the esophagus, stomach, small intestine, large intestine (also known as the colon), sigmoid colon, rectum and anus. We consume food and nutrients in the mouth, chew them, mix them with saliva, swallow them, and digest and absorb the nutrients from them over time. The fiber resists digestion and proceeds through to the end (and makes for bulkier stools that are easier to pass).

The intestine consists of both smooth (vascular) muscle and striated (skeletal) muscle, which work together to propel food along by a process called peristalsis. This explains why you can stand on your head and still digest food, although I cannot recommend it. The striated muscles are strikingly similar to the skeletal muscles that you use to move your body parts. The smooth muscle is similar to the blood vessel lining.

There are two orientations of gross gut muscles: concentric and longitudinal. The concentric, in effect, squeezes the chyme (food, water, digestive enzymes) along the tract and is neurologically synchronized with the longitudinal muscles. This synchronization by the intrinsic nervous system of the gut tells the muscles to move the chyme along, toward its storage in the rectum. If your nervous system is intact, and your incredible brain has its way, you can wait until it's opportune to deposit the waste in the toilet bowl. How amazing are we?!

With resistance exercise, these muscles become stronger and more efficient at doing their everyday work. Fiber exercises the muscles of the colon. It makes the GI tract muscles work harder, but it also makes them healthier in the process.

Fatty and carbohydrate-loaded meals do not require the same GI muscle exercise and can lead to a process of muscle weakening and thinning called atrophy. This atrophy directly leads to diseases such as diverticulosis and later, diverticulitis, and indirectly contributes to the development of hemorrhoids. Wow!

Dietary fiber, both soluble and insoluble, increases the speed at which the food travels through the GI tract, decreasing transit time. The shorter the time that fats, sugars, and toxic irritants remain in the system, the less likely they are to cause damage or predispose individuals to cancer. Fiber helps to decrease transit time and "clean up the human house interior." This minimizes the risk of colon cancer and makes the intestinal walls strong and healthy.

Is this easy, or what? Learn to minimize your intake of saturated fats, cholesterol, starch, and sugar. Then, maximize intake of fiber. This will give you a healthy inside and outside and a sense of well-being.

Earlier, we discussed the essential requirement for adequate daily water intake. Fiber alone will not move along smoothly, so it requires copious amounts of water to exert its helpful effects throughout your system. In review, it is recommended that a healthy person should consume 4 to 6 liters (approximately 1.5 gallons) of clean water daily. Some of this water is already present in the food we eat, such as vegetables, fruit, and non-caffeinated low-sugar beverages. Supplementing your diet with adequate amounts of water helps to flush waste products out of your body's organs. It ensures that all your body cells have the clean water they (and you !) need to survive.

The final word is exercise, believe it or not. It takes three things to "move your bowels." Exercise moves and strengthens your skeletal muscles. This not only moves body fluids around but also strengthens your respiratory and pelvic diaphragm, essential in pushing out waste feces. Water, fiber, and exercise are the three key elements to moving and grooving in the bathroom.

Increasing Fiber / Decreasing Constipation
Dietary Choice

<u>Grains:</u>

brown rice (1 cup long grain) – 3 g, oat bran (1 cup) – 7g, oatmeal (1 cup) – 5g, wheat bran (1 cup) – 25g, raisin bran (1 cup) 5g, whole wheat bread (1 slice) – 2g

<u>Vegetables:</u>

asparagus (8 large) – 2g, broccoli (1 cup) – 4g, carrots (1 cup) – 4g, corn(1 cup whole kernel) – 8g, potatoes(1 large) – 4g, squash (butternut) – 7g

Beans:

kidney beans (1 cup) – 15g, pinto beans (1 cup) – 20g, black-eyed peas (cup) – 16g, soy beans (1 cup dried) – 6g

Fruits:

prunes (5 dried) – 3g, raspberries (1 cup) – 6g, apple (with skin) – 3g, avocado (1 large) – 8g, cherries (1 cup pitted) – 2g

Supplements:

Chia seeds can be added to may foods
Psyllium seed fiber (Metamucil, etc.)
Fiber powder for drink mix
Fiber wafers and capsules
Methyl cellulose (Citrucel, etc.)

Drink 4-6 glasses of water per day

Dairy: Body fuel or inflammation fuel?

Is dairy #realfood? Here are a few answers you will hear to that question. "We need the calcium that milk supplies… It supplies necessary vitamin D… We've been drinking it forever, of course, it is good for you." The U.S. Dairy association advertised it for many years with, "Milk, it does a body good," and, "Got Milk?"

I believe and advocate that cow's milk (bovine milk secretion) is for calves (baby cows). Human milk is for baby humans. Additionally, the human body does not necessarily absorb calcium well from milk. Humans don't necessarily digest milk sugar (lactose) or milk protein (casein) well.

The dairy industry and large agribusinesses operate factory farms to produce milk by infusing their cows with steroids and antibiotics, using any means to increase product output and profits. The agribusiness industry supplements vitamin D into the product in lesser amounts and falsely claims it is in sufficient supply to have health benefits. The USDA, which we thought served as a regulatory agency, but never a nutrition entity, has become the marketing arm of the dairy agribusiness industry. Their "milk, it does a body good" claim is utterly (perhaps, "ud-derly") without merit, in my opinion.

Many adults are lactose intolerant and are made to feel that this is a disease that needs treatment. Nothing could be further from the truth. We lack the enzyme to break down lactose, and many of us have a tough time digesting casein/milk protein, because it is not a natural food for humans. Cheese and butter are much worse, as they are coagulated, artificially concentrated, dairy-saturated fat derivatives. Sorry, ice cream fans, cream and white sugar are #notfood either.

Dairy products can cause inflammation throughout the entire body, including inflammation of blood vessels. People with seasonal allergies often notice that their allergies, triggered by inflammatory reactions to pollen, cats, and other allergens, worsen when they consume dairy products.

Dairy, including milk, cream, cheese, cream cheese, yogurt, butter, and other derivatives of cow milk, is not quality human food, in my opinion. There are rare exceptions to every rule. If a person is allergic to many other food products, for whatever reason, dairy may become necessary. In my opinion, though, it is not an ideal food for most people.

Dr. Wax's Sensible Diet Choices

Avoid:	Instead:
Soda/Cola	Water
White bread/rolls	Whole Wheat Bread=3g fiber/slice
Potatoes/pasta	Spaghetti squash, zucchini pasta
White sugar	Honey
Candy	Fruit
Grapes, watermelon	Pear, apple, grapefruit, orange
Sugar ("kid's") cereals	Fiber cereals/bran
Pancakes/waffles	Oatmeal
Apple or cranberry juice	Fresh grapefruit or orange juice
Red meat	Fish
Pork/bacon/sausage	Tofu
Shellfish	Fish (salmon, tuna, etc.)
Fats (butter)	Unsaturated oils (olive)
Whole eggs/yolks	Egg whites
Whole milk	Soy, almond or rice milk
Cheese (high fat)	Soy Yogurt (low fat)
Canned Foods	Fresh foods

Other hints: Avoid eating after 7:00 PM

Have a healthy breakfast, lunch, and dinner
Drink plenty of water – 4-6 glasses of 8 oz. per day
Don't forget to exercise – 60 minutes per day
Think of pasta and potatoes as white, processed sugar – use sparingly

Here is a quick meal idea: Open a can of tuna or salmon and add it to a fresh vegetable salad.

Chapter Eleven
Sleep

"Sleep is the golden chain that ties health and our bodies together."

– Thomas Dekker

Sleep is an essential part of the human experience; growth, repair, energy regeneration. Sleep allows the body and mind to rest and reorganize. It allows for integration and "filing," of daily added information. The human body continuously cycles through a circadian rhythm, characterized by the wake-sleep cycle. Disturbances in sleep cause and worsen many medical problems. Therefore, it is essential to establish a regular, healthy sleep pattern.

Different people need different lengths of sleep. Some individuals require eight hours of sleep per night, while others are perfectly content with five. As we age, we generally require less sleep because our bodies grow less. It is an imperfect art to figure out how much any person needs at any stage of their life. Everyone, however, needs enough regular sleep to feel rested when they wake up and live out their daily activities.

There are many different causes of sleep disturbances. Sometimes it is hard to fall asleep. Other times, it is hard to stay asleep. Still other times, we awaken prematurely and cannot return to sleep, especially when strongly desired.

Sleep apnea is becoming increasingly common. Sleep

apnea is characterized by multiple extended moments of stopping breathing while asleep. We see it increasingly in the developed world as we become more obese. Obesity is the "largest" risk factor, pun intended of course, for obstructive sleep apnea. Usually, in my practice, the patient's spouse makes the diagnosis for me with observation of and complaints about the patients sleep; snoring and extended periods without breathing, punctuated by snorts and jerky body movements, like restless legs, as a response to the buildup of carbon dioxide and the lack of oxygen.

Commonly, people use their smartphones, tablets, smart watches, and computers multiple times during the day and for more extended periods than anticipated. The bright light from the device tells the brain that the day is not over. The body will not be ready for sleep and maintain proper sleep cycles for those people, especially those who use these devices close to bedtime.

There are many changes you can make to improve your sleep:

I. Improve your sleep environment.

    A. Keep your bedroom slightly cool.

    B. Keep your bedroom dark when going to sleep.

    C. Only use the bedroom to sleep. Do not use it for daytime activities.

    D. Avoid smartphone, tablet and computer use at least one hour before bedtime.

II. Adopt a healthy lifestyle to improve sleep.

    A. Avoid tobacco smoking and other stimulants.

    B. Avoid caffeine, a stimulant.

C. Avoid alcohol before bed.

D. Exercise regularly during the day, but not too close to bedtime.

E. Relax for a half-hour before going to bed to sleep.

F. Consider meditation, Yoga, breathing techniques, soothing music before bed.

G. Avoid daytime naps.

H. Do not go to bed until you begin to become sleepy.

I. Keep your body at a healthy weight;

J. Avoid obesity.

Sleep is a vital part of our daily lives and is crucial to our overall health. Follow the above recommendations, and you should improve your sleep/wake cycle. If you still have difficulty over a few nights a week or more, consult your family physician.

Chapter Twelve
Exercise Health

"The hardest thing about exercise is to start doing it. Once you are exercising regularly, the hardest thing is to stop it."

–Erin Gray

Oh, no! Exercise? Not that again.

"I don't have time for exercise in my daily routine. I go to work all day and am worn out when I get home. When am I supposed to exercise?"

"My children and their school, where I volunteer, takes up all of my time. Then, keeping the house clean and straight, and we can't afford a cleaner just so I have NO TIME to exercise."

"My back is killing me, my feet hurt, and I am worn out all the time."

Have you ever heard others use these excuses, or have you used them yourself? Do they sound familiar? They should, as they are pretty common. To some, they are reasons why not, but to me, they are excuses. I tell patients that I hear excuses all day long, every day, but I don't pay them any attention. Do you still believe all of your own (BS) excuses? Would you tolerate those same excuses from another seeking your experienced counsel?

Exercise is so vital to your body's health that it is not only possible, but critical to make time for it every day.

Some people, including the artist formerly known as "young me," dreaded exercise. In grade school and high school, I did my best to avoid any type of exercise. I remember thinking that the purpose of school was education. Gym class had nothing to do with worthwhile learning, in my opinion, at the time. It only distracted from that solitary education mission. Any time I could get a pass to do a project, or help a teacher, I would, "exit, stage left!"(as Snaggletooth/Snagglepuss would say in Hanna-Barbera's The Quick Draw McGraw Show, 1959). I avoided unnecessary movement. How could any U.S. President issue an award for gym exercise? Shouldn't they be rewarding intelligence, independence, and creative thinking instead?

Learning is necessary for the mind and life itself. Exercise also benefits the body in multiple ways, including increasing longevity and overall quality of life.

There are three fundamentally distinct types of exercise: stretching, cardiovascular (aerobic), and resistance (anaerobic), also known as weight (lifting) training. They are all essential for maintaining good health. Together, they can add years to your life and, perhaps even more importantly, quality to your years.

Exercise can make someone more physically attractive, while also adding to their confidence and self-esteem. It helps to keep a fresh supply of water constantly moving and recycling itself (as discussed in the water chapter). Life is motion, and motion is life. One of many things that differentiates us from furniture is our ability to move at will (among others).

Exercise is vital to our overall health and well-being. It can help protect you from various diseases, such as heart disease, stroke, hypertension, diabetes, and cancer, just to name a few.

Most Americans have become self-imposed victims of a sedentary lifestyle, i.e., they do not move around or exercise enough. This alone can prevent a person from achieving their optimal health. To be our best, we must prioritize time for exercise and other healthy lifestyle practices.

People exercise on a categorical scale, in my opinion. It can be broken down into distinct categories (1-5). We can compare the body to a car analogy. Here's my simple model for understanding your level of activity with its incumbent risks and benefits:

HINO Activity Levels

Class 1. Sedentary. In this group, people remain at rest from sunrise to sunset. Their work and daily activities are minimal. Their bodies don't need to respond to physical challenges, so they lose the capacity. If they were a car, they would sit out on the street in the rain, rusting solid (dying).

Class 2. Active. In this group, people are busy doing mildly strenuous activities, like steps, throughout the day. They will not have any volitional planned exercise but will be moving about with the activities of daily living (ADLs). This car is used a few times a week for short trips, but has a minor risk of corrosion (cancer), rather than rusting solid (death).

Class 3. Regular Exercise. In this group, people have set aside time for regular exercise, perhaps three to five times per week. They generally schedule and attend exercise sessions. This car runs well and only needs only routine maintenance and occasional repairs.

Class 4. Daily Exercise. These people are "religious" about their exercise; they are committed to it. They exercise daily and seldom miss a workout or spontaneous walk, bike, swim or run. This car is the most efficient, gets good mileage, and has excellent longevity, all in context.

Class 5. Endurance Exercise (Athletes). These people train daily and push extremely hard at regularly scheduled challenging events. They expect, enjoy, and practice maximal mental and physical challenges. One could argue that they are "addicted" to their events. They suffer more injuries and wear-and-tear than others. This car is driven "hard," frequently needs repair, and is at increased risk of breakdown.

My goal and practice is to stay in Class 4, where the most benefit meets the lowest disease risk. I also recommend it as a goal for many patients. Even those who are in Class 1 are sedentary and rusting in place. We must set aggressive yet achievable goals and track their progress. I ask those in a patient's support system to commend them as they achieve their objectives. They learn to ask and answer the question, "What am I worth?"

Stretching, cardiovascular, and resistance training work together to increase your vitality, stamina, and overall well-being.

Aerobic exercise primarily strengthens the cardiovascular (heart and blood vessel) system. This is achieved through various activities, including walking, jogging, running, rowing, cycling, swimming and other aerobic exercises. It is a pattern of physical activity that increases heart rate and breathing for a sustained period and relies on oxygen to generate energy for this activity.

A healthy target heart rate is 80% of your maximum heart rate (i.e., 220 minus your age in years). Aerobic exercise is best done daily, but exercising every other day (3-4 times a week) will also be beneficial. Aerobic exercise contributes to weight loss and also helps maintain a healthy weight. It will increase endurance and make you feel more vital and alive.

Resistance training involves lifting progressively more weight with your muscles. Usually, it consists of three or four sets of 10 repetitions of an exercise. This can be done three times per week, resistance training results in shapely muscles, increased strength, and more efficient muscle function.

Together, cardiovascular (aerobic) and resistance training can go a long way in helping prevent disease. It can also make you feel your best.

Best Use

So, how can I use these to my best advantage? I'm glad that you asked. First, start with a daily 10-minute stretching regimen. It should be done when you wake up in the morning, or at least before exercising. It should comprise stretching and mobility exercises for all major muscle groups. This will help you prepare for the day and any upcoming exercise. It will also help prevent injury.

Resistance training will improve your body's muscle function and appearance. It will help increase strength and give you a toned appearance. It is repetitive exercise with weights, resistance machines, or devices that allow your muscles to pull or push against resistance. Typically, three sets of 10 repetitions are performed to fatigue the muscle and signal it to grow. Each body part should be worked on at least once a week. For example, a sample regimen might include chest and triceps on day one, back and biceps on day two, legs and abdominals on day three, and so on. Once you get rolling, you can add other exercises that work the same muscles from different angles. You'll find that the body quickly habituates and acclimates to stressors, so you must vary the stressors for best fitness.

Cardiovascular exercise is arguably the most important for good health. It enhances your endurance and overall health. It entails activities such as brisk walking, jogging, (bi)cycling, running, and rowing for at least 30 minutes each day. Use the "good sweat rule" to determine if the activity is intense enough for the desired benefits. During the activity, you should get up a "good sweat," but still should be able to hold a brief conversation without totally losing your breath. This rule can be used to estimate that your target heart rate is approximately attained. Here is an example for a 40-year-old: 0.80 x (220-40) =144.

In addition to increased heart rate, breathing rate and sweating, your kidneys will work faster to process wastewater. This is increased glomerular filtration rate. You'll find, if you haven't already, that highly aerobic and cardiovascular exercise fills up your bladder quickly. Have you ever heard the phrase, "I've got to pee like a racehorse?" Well, now you understand why, when and how.

Look around. Those who walk daily seem to live longer and be more vital every day. This is no accident. Cardiovascular walking improves circulation, strengthens leg muscle tone, and promotes a general sense of wellness.

Perhaps you have heard that swimming in a pool is an excellent form of exercise. Unlike walking, it is a non-weight-bearing activity. This is a blessing and a curse. Those of us with "bad," meaning chronically painful, feet, knees, and hips, will appreciate swimming for that reason. Others, however, would benefit from weight-bearing exercises on their legs because it has been shown to decrease the likelihood of osteoporosis, or age-related bone thinning. Swimming also uses your arms and legs in motion, while walking is primarily a lower extremity exercise. Wouldn't it be nice to combine the best of both worlds? You're way ahead of me!

Swim walking combines the best and most beneficial aspects of swimming and walking in one inexpensive and fun exercise. All it requires is a good pair of walking, running, or cross-training shoes. It is walking with a twist. The twist is what makes it better than simply conventional walking.

Augment walking with two simple additions to make it swim-walking. First, begin walking at a moderate pace to follow the "good sweat rule;" walk quickly enough to get up a good sweat but still be able to hold a simple conversation at the same time. The only people this may be difficult for are those who cannot walk and chew gum.

Second, begin to turn your head to the left with each step. Next steps return your head to looking forward. Next step, look to your right. Then return to the center and repeat the process. This simple addition will strengthen your neck rotator muscles, increase your flexibility, decrease your stress, and help keep you safe from oncoming traffic.

Once you've mastered these simple steps of swim-walking, you've increased your efficiency and will reap more results from the exercise. Then you will want to add to your swimming time and strokes. Add the American crawl stroke. For non-swimmers, this means rotating your arms in large circles while walking, first in a forward direction. Later, advanced exercisers can add a backstroke to the technique. Alternating strokes and head motion can help decrease the possibility of boredom by mixing things up.

Swim-walking involves all four limbs and increases the number of calories you burn during exercise. The weight-bearing aspect will help build healthy bones in the spine and legs. This simple and enjoyable exercise will enhance the quality of your daily life and maximize your life potential.

Cardiovascular and resistance exercise is beneficial in improving the quality and quantity of your life (in years!). Stretching should precede and conclude all workouts, ideally. Consult with your family physician before starting any exercise program to ensure a safe start. Vary your workouts to avoid boredom!

Exercise – Yoga, Pilates, Aerobic classes, cycling, running, rowing, swimming, resistance training, etc.

Although all varieties of exercise benefit people, specific individuals may derive more benefits from some types than others. As we age, our bodies change. Further, with passing years, especially if we don't exercise often, our body tissues stiffen. Our muscles weaken and atrophy, while our bones lose density. This results in a greater risk of injury. Furthermore, our balance homeostasis weakens by our 60s and may result in chronic dizziness, making our daily efforts more challenging.

Yoga is beneficial as we age to maintain flexibility, strength, balance, and optimal health. Yoga is an ancient practice that enables practitioners to learn and grow throughout life, resisting the adverse effects of aging.

Joseph Pilates, who was chronically ill in his youth, invented Pilates in the early 1900s to strengthen the core muscles of the body. The core consists of the chest, abdomen, back, pelvis, and sacrum. Special emphasis is placed on the abdominal and pelvic diaphragms, which other types of exercise may miss. Anyone who takes a Pilates class will soon come to a new-found respect for the pelvic muscles!

Aerobic classes are so named because participants move quickly in a studio setting, exercising with others. They engage in whole-body cardiovascular exercise. The classes vary in intensity, duration, program, music, and many other variables. Aerobic classes are extremely popular at gyms and health clubs due to their variety. Teacher differences and class scheduling may positively or negatively be limiting factors.

Cycling is a wonderful way to exercise and appreciate the natural beauty of landscapes, flora, and fauna. The cyclist enjoys sunrises and sunsets that others miss; they're breathtaking in their beauty and enjoyed while improving one's health. There are many types of cycling, including road, mountain, cyclocross, and others.

Whether you're a beginner or expert, a visit to your local bike shop can be eye-opening. A cycling professional will guide you through all the options and tailor your bike choice to your body proportions. This is a massive advantage over big-box department and online stores, although it is usually more costly.

For those of us with neck and back issues (pretty much all those bipedal humans walking upright), recumbent bikes and trikes have a more relaxed seating position. These have alternative, non-traditional seating positions, taking the stress off the back and neck. These recumbent bikes require practice and sometimes determination to ride correctly and effortlessly, just as your first diamond frame bike did when you were six years old. There are even front-wheel-drive recumbent (Cruzebike) bikes to complement the common typical rear-wheel chain-driven bike. The choices of bikes, positions, and gear are as varied as the healthy people who ride them.

For inclement weather or personal preference, there is an indoor "spinning" cycling option. These distinctive stationary bikes differ from their traditional counterparts. They are engineered to duplicate the feel of outdoor cycling. The wheel of a spin bike is weighted down at 20lbs usually. This causes the rider to push against inertia to get it to move and keep it moving, which feels similar to outdoor cycling. In a spin class, the teacher calls out varying cycling positions as driving music plays in the background. This will stimulate your brain and help keep your legs and feet moving. Your heart rate and respiratory rate will join your speeding feet on their way to a healthier place.

Like all forms of exercise, running has both risks and benefits. We have all met "runners," totally devoted to the sport; live to run and run to live. They run miles daily and participate in marathons on weekends. You will find many adrenaline junkies in this exercise discipline. Running is a cardiovascular exercise that combines weight-bearing activity with loading of the axial joints. Runners develop excellent cardiovascular fitness, an athletic, slender physique, and increased bone density in their lower extremities. The sad news is that when running is overdone on manmade solid road surfaces, the knees, hips, and ankles can wear out by age 50. This is why I'm not a personal fan of running, although I respect its goals and devotees. It is crucial to find the right running shoes at a local private running store. Additionally, consider consulting a trainer and sports physician or podiatrist to help guide your safe and effective transition into this addictive sport.

Rowing is a great exercise that emphasizes both muscle strength and cardiovascular fitness, depending on the resistance and speed of the row. It uses the back and biceps muscles while extending the legs, engaging those muscles as well.

Outdoor rowing is the pinnacle of this activity. You don't always have a boat and a body of water handy or available. Many home rowing machines recreate this exercise in different ways. The classic rowing machine, since about 1980, has been using a seat that slides, a rowing bar that pulls a bicycle chain, and a fan wheel. The fan wheel provides resistance to exercise. Other models employ alternative methods, such as a paddle that moves in a circular motion through a tank of water. Most models will provide decades of use.

Of course, one must mention lap swimming as one of nature's near-perfect exercises. It is a non-weight-bearing exercise that uses most muscle groups and incorporates cardiovascular exercise with resistance training. People are buoyant (float) in the water which takes pressure off the spine and axial joints like knees and hips. Swim lessons that teach water safety, comfort, and various strokes in early childhood are a terrific lifelong gift to give any child. Are you listening, grandparents?

Chapter Thirteen
Considerations & Other Healthy Choices

"Osteopathy is based on the perfection of Nature's work. When all parts of the human body are in line we have health. When they are not the effect is disease. When the parts are readjusted disease gives place to health."

–Andrew Taylor Still, DO

Inflammation

Inflammation is a common element in most human diseases. Most people think of the immune system, lymphatic system, and circulatory system as a defense against foreign intruders, such as viruses and bacteria. Well, it's much more incredible than that.

Andrew Taylor Still, DO, recognized the body's innate ability for self-maintenance and repair in about 1874. Since that time, medical research, science, and physician practice have discovered many mechanisms of the body. The key uniting and common element is inflammation.

Think of inflammation as a building wrecking crew, highly skilled and trained to take apart and remove non-functional or malfunctioning elements. To build new buildings and structures, the old, outdated, broken, or even dangerous ones must be carefully removed. This clears the way for new, useful, and effective ones. Our body removes and replaces elements that will harm us every moment of every day. It not only defends us against intruders from without but also against invaders from within, like cancer cells. The immune system is constantly surveilling our cells to ensure we maintain good cell health.

The immune system is both military and police forces. It acts as the military to defend the body borders against invading pathogens. It also acts as police force to remove deviant cells, like cancer cells, from within, as discussed above. It learns to recognize new threats as they occur, both at the borders and in the deepest recesses. How amazing is our immune system?

You have cancer. What?! Yes, I said it. Sorry. So do I. What am I saying? Every living person has cancerous cells within them. If so, then why don't we get sick and die? Our immune system destroys and removes these cells before they can establish themselves. Occasionally, some cancer cells get out of hand and a person develops "cancer," but this is rare, given the absolute number of cancerous cells and the frequency at which they occur in our bodies. This is why daily health is so important. And, your approach to good health must be consistent in every waking moment.

Maximizing your health with all the best lifestyle choices is a constant battle. You can think of it as the classic struggle of good versus evil, or man versus nature.

Inflammation is the bodily process that breaks you down to build you up. It must remain in balance. If you are breaking down more cells than building new ones, you become ill. If you are building more healthy cells than you're breaking down, or at least keeping up, you feel vital and energized.

Not only can viral and bacterial invaders cause inflammation, but so-called foods can also trigger inflammation. When your body encounters these "food insults" repeatedly, you get chronic inflammation that results in chronic disease—yet another reason to be diligent and persistent in your healthy food choices. Symptoms such as fever and coughing can be indicative of this inflammation battle. Symptoms such as fatigue, lack of concentration, dizziness, sleeplessness, and other constitutional symptoms may indicate that the inflammation battle rages within you because of poor lifestyle choices. Concentrated sugars and saturated fats are notorious for increasing the inflammation cascade.

Poisons like smoke, whether tobacco, cannabis, or other products, increase body inflammation and can damage your DNA. In other words, smoke can cause cancer in every organ in your body. Although people think of smoking as causing lung cancer, all other cancers also occur more frequently in smokers, even skin cancer.

So, other than avoiding eating, drinking, and exposing yourself to inflammation-provoking things, how can you reduce inflammation? Glad you asked. A well-hydrating vegetable-based diet is a critical staple in a healthy lifestyle.

Daily exercise helps reduce overall cellular and body inflammation, particularly through cardiovascular exercise. Exercise initially increases inflammation but eventually will result in an overall reduction in inflammatory body processes. This is key to best health and longevity.

Skin Health

Skin "age spots," as they are commonly called, are not related to skin age. They are the result of permanent damage to the skin caused by cumulative sun and other ultraviolet (UV) light exposure, especially when exposed in tanning beds. Sun damage accumulates over the years and is exacerbated by blistering sunburns and prolonged sun exposure.

Sun exposure causes numerous changes in skin color and texture over time. It causes wrinkling, thinning of the skin, and other cosmetic issues. Skin cancer is the most common form of cancer in the United States. More than two million skin cancers are diagnosed annually in the U.S.

Keratoses, or brown spots, such as seborrheic and actinic, can alter the color and texture of some regions of the skin surface. Seborrheic keratosis is a benign skin change often confused with actinic. Actinic keratosis is a pre-cancerous lesion induced by UV sun exposure. These are a warning to reduce your sun exposure and protect yourself with clothes, shade, and sunblock.

Basal cell carcinoma (read that as cancer) is a superficial skin layer cancer that can be removed in its entirety, once detected, by a physician. It spreads slowly over months to years by direct extension, not metastasis.

Squamous cell carcinoma, if large enough, tends to go deeper into the skin and may have a metastatic risk over time.

Malignant melanoma is, by far, the worst because it can be small and virulent, spreading more quickly by metastasis to other body organs. It has the highest risk of recurrence and metastatic spread by far. It can be deadly if not prevented, detected, or treated early. It is, indeed, "the Sword of Damocles."

What can be done to protect yourself against such potentially awful skin diseases? I'm glad that you asked. Preventive skin care is our primary defense against these maladies. The good news is that it is easy to protect your skin by avoiding sun damage. No tanning by the sun or tanning beds is safe. Avoid unnecessary exposure, especially during the peak hours of 10:00 AM to 3:00 PM in all seasons. The skin should be covered with clothing, such as long sleeves and hats with wide brims. Apply sunblock with a sun protection factor (SPF) of 50 to the face, arms, and any other exposed areas before going outside.

A simple rule of thumb is "slip, slop, and slap." This program helped reduce the skin cancer rates in Australia, which were epidemic in the 1990s. Slip on a shirt. Slop on sunblock of SPF 50 and slap on a wide-brimmed hat to reduce your risk.

Sunglasses with UV protection and polarization will go a long way in preserving your eyesight. It will help prevent cataracts from forming as your eyes age. Wrap-around sunglasses do the best job of filtering the light from most angles.

In my opinion, mineral based sunblock with titanium dioxide and/or zinc oxide physical blockade outperforms chemical sunscreens in reducing UV exposure, sunburn, and cancer risk. I prefer a combination of both in my sunblock, rather than just chemical sunscreen.

These techniques will enable you to take control of your skin health and prevent unsightly and potentially harmful issues. Do you want proof? Look at how smooth and silky your skin is on the non-sun-exposed areas, i.e., below the belt line. With proper skin care throughout your life, it is possible to maintain beautiful and healthy skin.

Prevention is the most effective tool for avoiding unsightly and potentially deadly skin damage.

Sexual health

A satisfying and safe sex life is essential to any healthy adult lifestyle. The issue of safe sex is paramount. These days, we cannot only prevent unplanned pregnancy but also prevent sexually transmitted infections (STDs/STIs). Why bother? It cannot affect me, can it?

STIs include the big newsmakers such as Human Immunodeficiency Virus (HIV), Acquired Immune Deficiency Syndrome (AIDS) to the less vogue diseases like herpes simplex virus (HSV), genital warts/human papilloma virus (HPV), and Chlamydia (no acronym abbreviation available yet).

There are "the classics," such as syphilis (treponema pallidum) and gonorrhea (Neisseria gonorrhoeae). Do they all still exist? Hasn't modern medicine done away with all these annoyances? The unfortunate answer to the former is yes, and the latter is no. They all exist in the quiet of people's bedrooms, even in senior citizen retirement communities and nursing homes, surprisingly enough.

Part of the problem is that most people are unaware of the signs and symptoms. Another part is that people do not think that it could happen to them for a variety of reasons. This plays a significant role in the rising incidence of these diseases in the teenage population; they are young, vibrant, and often perceive themselves as invincible. In real life, however, we are all subject to these problems if we choose not to protect ourselves and our partners.

Maybe you have heard it all before: Abstinence is the only sure method of sexually transmitted disease prevention and birth control. True. But it is possible to protect yourself and minimize your risk and still retain a "good sex life." Maybe you have also heard the monogamy speech. It is a helpful part of the plan to stay healthy. If you are not planning for disease prevention and pregnancy prevention, you are planning for disaster.

Safe sex techniques stress monogamous behavior and barrier methods of birth control. Barrier methods refer to the male and female condoms. These two devices (devices?) minimize the skin and secretion exposure for both partners. Of course, masturbation in private setting has zero risk of STIs, but please (!), do not attempt in public.

Although at the time of writing, female condoms are available but still under testing for pregnancy and disease transmission prevention data. I believe that they are more effective in disease prevention than their male condom counterparts. Properly used (yes, it takes a mite more effort), it covers more of the areas in contact. All sexually active people, outside a long-term mutually monogamous relationship, should use barrier methods of birth control, like male and female condoms. The life you save may be your own or your partner's!

Consider the deadly STI called AIDS, caused by HIV, human immunodeficiency virus. Whether we are major media stars, sports figures, musicians, drug users, hookers/sex workers, homosexuals, heterosexuals, men, women, children, high school students, college students (more "invincibles" there!), whites, blacks, Asians, Hispanics, middle-easterners, and any other ethnic background, we are all vulnerable to HIV. You are at risk. You can't see it, smell it, taste it, or feel it, so protect yourself from it.

The less glamorous STIs are still a problem.

Herpes is a virus that, once you contract it, becomes a lifelong companion. Sores break out now and again, and they itch and weep. Yes, we have medicine to minimize attacks, but it cannot be cured. The HSV virus is also likely responsible for "fever blisters" and "canker sores" that recur in your mouth and on your lips.

Two types of the Herpes Simplex virus are currently understood: type I and type II (pretty straightforward). Type I usually occurs in the mouth and on the lips. Don't panic! More than 90% of the population by age 65 experiences an oral virus. It is endemic—it lives within our population.

Type II Herpes is more commonly associated with the genital area. It causes similar sores to occur episodically in the groin and on the genitals. This variety spreads through sexual contact.

Yes, it is possible to get HSV type I on your genitals. It is also possible to get HSV type II in your mouth (I think the mode of spread is obvious here—oral sex). This sort of thing begs us to be smart and use common sense about safe sex practices to prevent permanent HSV infection.

Like its cousin, chicken pox virus (herpes zoster virus), HSV stays recessed in the dorsal root ganglia of infected nerves. Your immune system is the police force that keeps it there, until it is disturbed. Then the virus follows the infected nerves to the skin surface to produce the characteristic ulcer lesions that hurt.

For those with HSV, consider L-Lysine 1,000mg daily on an empty stomach to help impede viral return to surface skin.

The HPV virus is responsible for genital warts and is also sexually transmitted. This virus, like HSV, also has no cure. The warts can be removed, but the virus will live on in other infected cells. The more problematic part is that it can cause cancer of the cervix in women. Again, it is best not to get it by utilizing safe sex techniques.

To recap, if you are going to indulge in sexual activity, do it in a low-risk, healthy way. Male and female condoms, as well as monogamous, long-term relationships, are tools to remain healthy and disease-free.

Signs and Symptoms

Signs and symptoms are your body's way of communicating with you. Pain is a signal you get when something is wrong, infected, disrupted or damaged in some way. The nervous system is designed to provide signals and progress reports. A classic example is the simple reflex arc, such as when you put your hand on a hot stove. In less than a second, your sensory nerve realizes that the hand is in danger if it stays where it is! The impulse is transmitted to your spinal cord, which sends a command to your motor nerves in your hand to move quickly. The impulse is sent to your brain so that you won't make that mistake again (hopefully).

Your body also has a more complicated reflex arc. It takes a few seconds longer to initiate. For example, consider crossing the street rather slowly. A car is heading toward you. You see it and perhaps hear the horn as well. Your brain interprets these visual and auditory signals and compares them with information stored in your brain. The decision is made to get out of the way and flee to safety.

Symptoms are the language that your body speaks. All you

have to do is listen and understand what they mean. Then, take appropriate action.

Vital Signs

You have heard of vital signs in medical offices, hospitals, and in entertainment programs. Nowadays, people are measuring their progress vicariously through "smart" devices like smart-phones, smartwatches, smart rings, and fitness trackers. Having a basic understanding of vital signs, or measurements of bodily functions, can provide you with valuable insight into your health.

Height and weight provide a general indication of whether your system is grossly (no pun intended this time) off track to run efficiently. Height is how tall you are. Medical experts have created and published charts that consider age, height, sex, and weight, comparing them to scientifically established norms. Body mass index (BMI) is a person's weight in kilograms divided by the square of height in meters. It can provide a thumbnail sketch as to whether you are of normal weight, overweight, or morbidly obese. A BMI below 18.5 is considered underweight, 18.5-24.9 is regarded as a healthy weight, 25.0-29.9 is considered over-weight, and a BMI over 30.0 is considered obese. BMI doesn't consider someone's heritage, ancestry, or individual frame. Some individuals will never be in the "green zone" on a government weight or BMI chart. Ultimately, each person's choices are the final determinant of a healthy weight and body habitus, not a chart. They are only for reference.

Respiratory rate is a simple measure that indicates whether you are experiencing respiratory distress. Assuming your body is not stressed, your respiration should be between 12 and 20 breaths per minute. When you exercise, your breathing rate can increase to around 30 breaths per minute, but it returns to normal at rest. If you have a high respiratory rate while you are sick or otherwise not feeling well, it's time to call your physician for an appointment or go to the Hospital emergency department (ER/ED) if your life is in danger.

Heart rate, also known as pulse rate, indicates how fast your heart is beating and how efficiently your body is perfusing. The heart beats to circulate oxygenated blood to all your tissues and remove waste products, such as carbon dioxide. The faster the heart beats per minute (BPM) and the pulse responds, the more excited the system is. A resting heart rate can range from 50 to 89 BPM; lower is generally better and more efficient. The heart rate with activity is usually over 90-160 BPM. These are general ranges because they vary from individual to individual.

The refinement of heart rate is a matter of rhythm. That refers to the timing of the heartbeats, whether they are in sync or out of sync with each other. First, is it a regular or irregular rhythm? Whether fast or slow, a rhythm is regular if there is the same length of pause between the beats. Second, a beat is irregular if the time between beats varies. Third, irregular is split into regularly irregular and irregularly irregular. Regularly irregular is like three beats, pause, three beats, pause (trigeminy). Irregularly irregular is the sound and feel of popcorn popping, all different length pauses between beats. The beat may even feel different, which is usually atrial fibrillation, and should be examined by a physician or the hospital emergency department immediately, if initial occurrence.

You can monitor a heart for basic functions and disturbances. To reiterate the opening disclaimer, these ideas, classifications, and techniques are provided for general informational and educational purposes and should not be considered medical advice.

Pain

Pain is likely the most frequent problem, or indicator of body dysfunction, which drives a patient to see a medical professional. Pain manifests itself in our daily living activities, interactions with others, and work. It is more than our car's check engine light, but a physically disruptive force that can disturb your mental and physical well-being.

There are many causes of pain. These include trauma, bleeding, infection, organ disruption, bone fracture, cancer, osteopathic somatic dysfunction, and others.

An ignored cause of head, back, and limb pain is fascial somatic dysfunction and scarring. Fascia is an amazing, flexible substance that invests and covers all internal organs, muscles, nerves, blood vessels, bones, and tissues. When the body gets hit with a force, or trauma, it responds acutely (immediately) and chronically (long-term), if not appropriately dealt with. Fascia is pushed and pulled in multiple directions. If not stretched out and corrected to form and function, it scars, pushes, and pulls for a lifetime, causing dysfunction and structural damage, even osteoarthritis, destruction of bones and joints.

Back Pain

Back pain is one of the leading causes of work absences in the United States. It is also a frequent reason for people to seek medical care. It can happen after a trauma like a car accident, a fall, restless sleep, or seem to come on spontaneously.

There are many diverse causes for back pain. Somatic dysfunction, muscle strains, and ligament strains are the most common. They can be treated simply with rest and gentle osteopathic manipulation. Stretching exercises can help a person return to normal and prevent further injuries. Cold or warm compresses can be applied. Also, pain-reducing medications and muscle relaxants can be used.

Some sources of pain are more serious and problematic to treat, like spinal stenosis, the narrowing of the spinal canal, which compresses the spinal cord. Severe kidney infection can also be responsible for intense back pain. Herniated disks in the spine can compress nerve roots, causing pain and numbness in some cases.

Heart disease (problems with the blood supply to the heart) can be responsible for mid-back, shoulder, neck, and jaw pain.

Lung infections and smoking can irritate the back muscles by producing a vigorous cough. Stomach, intestinal, and gallbladder problems can also cause back pain.

If you suffer regular pain or experience sudden pain, you must see a physician about these problems if they do not resolve quickly. Osteopathic physicians (D.O.) have special training in the diagnosis and treatment of the musculoskeletal system (muscles, bones, fascia, ligaments, tendons, lymph, and blood vessels, etc.). Chiropractors (D.C.) and physical therapists (PT, MPT, DPT, alternately known as physiotherapists), also overlap in training and skills in this area but are limited in scope from medicine and surgery.

Maintaining proper posture, adopting a healthy lifestyle, and engaging in regular exercise are key to preventing back injuries and avoiding back pain.

Chest pain

Chest pain can be a symptom of various health issues, the most common of which is somatic dysfunction. This is a medical term that describes conditions involving muscles, nerves, fluids, and bones, which may result in pain. The muscles may be strained. The nerves may be extra-excitable; the blood and lymph may be restricted in their flow. The bones may not be moving correctly, or there may be inflammation at the joints (costochondritis). All these problems may exist separately or together to produce pain.

Chest pain is a common symptom, as it is associated with numerous health problems and diseases. These may include diseases and dysfunction of the heart, lungs, esophagus, stomach, gallbladder, rib cage, chest muscles, back muscles, and shoulder muscles, among others. It is the physician's job to determine the cause of chest pain and prescribe appropriate treatment.

Some causes of chest pain may be life-threatening, such as a heart attack. Others may not be as critical, such as pneumonia.

A patient's health history, combined with a physical exam and laboratory tests, allows a physician to determine the problem and how to address it.

Many symptoms, when coupled with chest pain, can indicate the cause. Shortness of breath or pain radiating to the left shoulder, back, or jaw can indicate the need for immediate medical attention. Cough, fever, lethargy, or belching is usually less severe but may still require attention. Heartburn pain can go either way. If it is related to exertion and accompanied by shortness of breath, it may be a medical emergency. If it is related to fatty food intake, smoking, or acidic food intake, it is not urgent but does require medical follow-up (and a lifestyle change).

In a large majority of cases, chest pain is the result of somatic dysfunction. A muscle strain in the chest, back, shoulder, or rib cage may be responsible. Although somatic dysfunction is not as serious as a heart attack, it may be confused with one, depending on how the patient feels, looks, and sounds. ("All chest pain is not angina," CM Wax, JAOA 1997). For this reason, your physician must be able to differentiate all the possible causes of chest pain. He or she must also be able to treat them.

Fever

A newborn's fever is the nemesis of any new mommy or daddy. It can strike fear into the heart of first-time parents. But we all get fevers from time to time. Is it urgent, or isn't it?

Television, radio, newspapers, magazines, the Internet, and other forms of media lead us to believe that fever is a problematic condition. Why? Most of them are funded by advertisers who sell drugs to reduce fever artificially. Additionally, allopathic (MD) , or conventional Western medicine aims to suppress symptoms, such as fever, in an attempt to alleviate the sickness; the absence of symptoms indicates the absence of disease, so it appears to some.

Fever is the human body's natural response to an invading pathogen, bacteria, virus, yeast, or other entity. It is not the body's attempt to self-destruct. The immune system, which constantly fights invaders (even as you read this book), works more effectively when the body temperature is slightly higher than usual (<98.6°F). With certain infections, the body seeks to enhance its performance to eradicate the invader. Fever is the body's response to increase immune system efficiency and maintain homeostasis.

The media is inundated with pharmaceutical advertisements promising to bring down fever quickly. Why? To sell products and make money. In most cases, these products are unnecessary and may even be counterproductive to your body's natural healing process. Fever alone is only dangerous when it is sustained over 103°F for a few days. It then begins to affect your hydration status more. Fever causes your body to lose water faster than at normal body temperature. Adults should ensure they drink an extra liter of water each day for every degree above 100°F. This will help avoid dehydration and support the body's natural processes.

Remember, fever is not an enemy. It is a friend. It alerts you to the fact that something is going on (a symptom). It enhances your immune system's efficiency in its fight. See your physician if you have a sustained fever for more than a few days.

If you're a child, a fever means you can stay home from school. That was only a joke, parents! Think back to your own experience of taking an occasional unplanned childhood day off.

Shortness of Breath

Feeling like you cannot catch your breath is a scary feeling. Most people take breathing for granted, as the body usually does a harmonious and continuous job of it. Shortness of breath can be a concerning sign that something is amiss.

The body does everything for a reason. Nothing occurs by chance. Despite this, we cannot always comprehend the reason. Sometimes, the reason may be as simple as running to catch a bus. Other times, it can be due to a heart or lung problem. Once again, we must be in touch with our body's system of signs and symptoms.

Shortness of breath can be a symptom of many different conditions. Asthma can cause an inability to catch your breath. It is a Reversible Airway Disease (RAD) that waxes and wanes. Removing allergens from your living and working space can help. These include dust, cats, dogs, perfumes, and other similar substances. It is readily treatable with prevention and inhaled medications, as recommended by a physician.

Chronic obstructive pulmonary disease (COPD) is a condition like asthma. It occurs with the lungs having a smaller functional area in which to perform their work of gas exchange. Most cases are caused by smoking tobacco products (cigarettes, cigars, and pipes). Only a few cases are of unknown cause. Because smoking is the predominant factor in the development of COPD, it is easy to avoid; do not smoke (it's that simple).

Respiratory infections can cause a cough and shortness of breath. These may include bronchitis, pneumonia, walking pneumonia, tracheitis, sinusitis, and others. With infective processes, a fever, thick sputum (mucus), and cough may be present.

Heart disease can also cause similar shortness of breath. One type, called Congestive Heart Disease (CHD), can mimic COPD or RAD. CHF can be life-threatening, so take it seriously and seek your physician if there are any questions.

The body is a great compensator. It has many mechanisms to manage stress. Suppose we remove ourselves or do not respond to the stressor; our body's message changes. In the absence of this stimulus, our breathing rate should slow down. If it does not occur in a reasonable and customary time frame or occurs frequently, your physician should evaluate it. He or she can help to "get to the bottom of it," and restore calm and confidence.

At every turn, our body communicates with us. We need only to lend an ear to listen.

Chapter Fourteen
The HINO Lifestyle
Prevention–Putting it all Together

"Praevenire est melius quam curare."
("Prevention is better than cure.")

– Desiderius Erasmus (1466-1536)

Like happiness, good health is a pursuit, not a state of being. Developing and maintaining healthy habits is an everyday, lifelong process. It is not a momentary project. As you have reached this point in the book, you may be feeling the weight and enormity of lifestyle changes. You may be wondering whether it is even possible. You are in luck. It is.

Every long journey begins with one step. You have taken the first step by reading this book and perhaps have taken other steps that have brought results in the past. Maybe what you tried before left you feeling orphaned because it did not produce the intended results. The habits with which you currently struggle are addictive in their effects. Your new life will combine several factors to slowly, incrementally, overcome the bad and replace it with the good.

A healthy diet, regular exercise, adequate hydration, quality sleep, relaxation, and effective time management are the antidote for your current struggles, and taken together, they are powerful tools to achieve your new health goals. Your Health Is Number One (HINO).

Here is an example of the HINO lifestyle: Start with a good night's sleep. Go to bed earlier, like 9 or 10 PM. Rise earlier, such as at 5 AM, and start a one-hour exercise program. For the first week or two, it will seem untenable, and your alarm clock will appear to be your mortal enemy, but it is not so. Ideally, optimal health begins after a complete night's sleep, accompanied by at least an hour of exercise in the early morning. There is even evidence to support that dawn's early light is healthy for your brain and state of health. Even Benjamin Franklin opined, "Early to bed and early to rise makes a man healthy, wealthy and wise," in Poor Richard's Almanac, in 1735 Philadelphia, Pennsylvania, United States.

After a month or so, your body may awaken without prompting at 5 AM if you have achieved 6-8 hours of sleep and your innate sleep cycles have completed themselves. Stretching should precede and follow the exercise routine to prevent injury. You may need to have a quick snack with water, such as an apple, before working out, especially for aerobic exercise. Others may only require water hydration. Either is OK, but a snack can follow exercise. Studies show that consuming real, healthy food eaten after exercise doesn't translate into weight gain but instead, provides the body with fuel and promotes muscle repair. Multiple controlled studies indicate that eating during or immediately after acute exercise typically does not result in compensatory overeating that nullifies the exercise benefit. In fact, subjects often maintain or improve the energy deficit created by exercise. That said, long-term weight effects depend on consistency, diet choices, and individual psychology.

After exercising, consider having a quick healthy snack, if necessary, attend to your hygiene routine: use the bathroom, shower, shave, brush your teeth, and so on. Get dressed for the activities of your day, whatever they may be. Enjoy a healthy breakfast with the family if possible. Your daily breakfast should be concluded in time for you to get your children on their buses or to take them to school.

"[Eat] Breakfast like a king, lunch like a prince, and dinner like a pauper," said Adelle Davis, the "first lady of nutrition." Her advice is wise. It tells us to break with the industrial revolution end-loaded food schedule that often ignores breakfast, indulges in carbs and a fatty lunch, then loads up on calories at supper.

Begin and practice a front-loaded eating schedule, where more food calories are consumed in the first half of the day than in the last half. This helps give your body ample time to utilize calories for energy and repair its cells. This is a healthy approach.

Quit storing calories as fat at the end of your day. Incidentally, that is the reason that big, heavy dinners followed by overwhelmingly caloric, fatty, sweet treats for dessert will result in obesity, morbidity (illness), and mortality (death).

It has been my longtime practice to rise at 5:00 AM, stretch, exercise, clean up, and eat a healthy breakfast. My goal is to be in my office by 9 AM.

Is this you?

Many people have clinical (detected) or subclinical (undetected) hypoglycemia, or low blood sugar, leading to fatigue, low energy, low motivation, brain fog, or daytime somnolence (sleepiness). Your new eating regimen can overcome all of these symptoms. Eat a small portion of healthy food three times during the workday. After breakfast at 7:30 AM, have a snack at 10:00 AM if necessary, lunch at noon, and a (non-carb) snack at 2:30 PM. If you have snacks, don't eat afternoon carbs as they may put you to sleep and add to weight gain. Try nuts, seeds, and legumes (beans) instead.

Be sure to take regular bathroom breaks to urinate and such. The body continuously generates urine throughout the day, and the night, for that matter. People, like teachers, are often made to feel that they must be in class from 8 AM to 3 PM without food or bathroom breaks. This leads to overeating after the workday and contributes to a higher incidence of urinary tract infections and problems due to excessive efforts at holding back urine during the workday. Health is number one; a healthy lifestyle prevents these bothersome issues.

Move around during your workday. Excessive sitting and standing in one place can be damaging to your joints, blood vessels and overall health in the long term. Movement, such as walking and changing positions frequently, can help avert these problems.

For those with desk jobs, here are some helpful tips. Ensure your desk or workstation is set up for optimal comfort and ergonomic efficiency. You'll feel better, and you'll produce consistently higher-quality work. Stretching, like rolling your shoulders around backward and forward, and stretching your neck from side to side, every ten to fifteen minutes, will help alleviate the "stress," muscle tension, headache, and neck ache that comes with taking work stress in a sedentary position.

If you have a family, use dinner as an opportunity to bond and enjoy quality time with your loved ones. Eat healthy vegetable-based meals. Avoiding excessive saturated fat and carbohydrate intake (sugar and starch). These will ultimately slow you down and sap your remaining energy for the remainder of the day. A lighter, predominantly vegetable-based diet will enhance your nutrition without hindering your work progress or encouraging weight gain. Two days a week, I return to work from 6:00 to 9:00 PM. A lighter dinner makes a major difference in my wakefulness and work performance for the late afternoon and early evening.

Upon return home from work, you may need an hour to "unwind." I know that I do, and my family recognizes it also and gives me that time—usually. Reading, chatting with family, listening to music, or catching up on snail mail (USMAIL) before your nighttime hygiene and bedtime routines will help you prepare for a restful night's sleep.

The Health Is Number One (HINO) lifestyle, detailed here, is a straightforward approach to programming your body for health and maintaining it. During this journey, you will fine-tune these new routines; they will become your own healthy habits.

Everyone has unique family situations, professions, jobs, likes, dislikes, and resources. The HINO lifestyle plan serves as a comprehensive guideline to provide a starting point for improving every aspect of your lifestyle, thereby contributing to your health and longevity journey.

Chapter Fifteen
The Meaning of Life

"The meaning of life is whatever you ascribe it to be."

–Joseph Campbell

This chapter on the meaning of life could, itself, be a book. A movie perhaps? Dr. Craig Wax's Meaning of Life (think Monty Python's The Meaning of Life-LOL). Adequately and thoroughly describing the meaning of life would fill a library. For the sake of brevity and perspective, I will be brief, although that may be difficult on many levels. After all, "Brevity is the soul of wit," wrote William Shakespeare in Hamlet.

Life is not about happiness, but purpose, meaningfulness, and expectations. It is a common misconception that life is all about pleasure and happiness. If that were the case, it would be about pleasure seeking 24/7 and accomplishing nothing. Noted psychologist Dr. Jordan Peterson speaks extensively about this in recent years.

- "Happiness is a pointless goal. Don't compare yourself with other people; compare yourself with who you were yesterday. Meaning is better than happiness."
- "The purpose of life is finding the largest burden that you can bear and bearing it."

- "It's in responsibility that most people find the meaning that sustains them through life."

Expectations play a key role in your effectiveness, happiness, and success. If you expect less and accomplish more, you tend to feel happier and more satisfied. If you expect more and accomplish less, you feel unhappy and dissatisfied. Setting your expectations is crucial to all your goals. Set moderate goals, including short-term, intermediate, and long-term objectives. If you set a huge goal, such as losing 100 pounds, you may feel overwhelmed and defeated before you start. Work on losing a pound a week or four to five pounds in a single month. In this way, you'll be more likely to meet your goals and remain mentally and physically energized to continue on your journey.

You set yourself up for disappointment if you choose a huge all-or-nothing proposition. Many diets, exercise plans, and lifestyle counsellors advocate days off and cheat days. On the contrary, I only advocate for success days, not cheating days. It's tough to get back on the proverbial "wagon" when you've disrupted your regular body chemistry function with the ingestion of non-food (#NotFood), taking a day off exercise, or the like. There will be errors, mistakes, and setbacks, all without you planning them! Stay on track, and you won't have to expend extra mental, emotional, and physical energy to get back on track. You will achieve more goals, happiness, and successes with a zero-tolerance policy for errors.

In my opinion, human nervous systems and biochemistry like to form habits, good or bad. Anything that stimulates certain neurotransmitters will become a subconscious goal for your body, whether it is beneficial or not. You want your neurotransmitters to align with the goals of your thought processes. This is the basis of the battle between the heart and the mind, Apollo versus Dionysus. I first learned about this in my four years of Latin class in high school (special thanks to the late Peter Aloysius Devlin, my Latin and English teacher). Mr. Devlin approved of the modern musical story adaptation by Neil Peart and Rush in Cygnus X-1,

Book II: Hemispheres, a progressive rock music staple of my youth.

We all have the capacity for reason and discipline. With "circumstances" (maybe another Rush song reference…), we all also face the pitfalls of dependence, addiction, and free-falls. Think of "yo-yo" dieting, concerning the simple toy that spins on a string, going up and down repeatedly. Yo-yos make good toys, but a lousy eating regimen. Take 100% control, challenging as it may be, to stay focused on your diet, exercise, and lifestyle. You're in charge all the time; 24x7x365.

Take on the HINO challenge! Optimize your health. Start walking, swimming, bicycling, or running. Attend to a healthy diet. Get an academic degree. Get a job. Start a business. Get married and have a child. Help people. Build something. Run for an organization, community, or government position.

"To finish the moment, to find the journey's end in every step of the road, to live the greatest number of good hours, is wisdom," wrote Ralph Waldo Emerson.

More simply put, in 1920, pastor Lynn Hough wrote, "Life is a journey and not a destination." To top it off, my wife added, "and there's no rush to the end."

There's, indeed, no end to the adventures and missions you could take on, just not necessarily simultaneously(!). Classic writers have written much about this. To recap: It's the journey, not the destination, and so on. Discover your path to meaning and bliss and get started.

Each journey begins simply with a mindset, a plan, and a single first step.

Chapter 16
Advance Directives

"Our prime purpose in life is to help others. And if you can't help them, at least don't hurt them."

–Dalai Lama

Advance directives are the rules that you wish others to follow in case you suffer a dire and potentially deadly health emergency. They inform physicians and other healthcare team members about what you would and would not want. These directives are helpful if your chances of meaningful survival are poor and you cannot communicate your wishes directly. The medical team is supposed to follow your advance directive. They are important because they speak for you when you cannot speak for yourself. Most states have default directives for those found down, unable to communicate, and with unknown resources.

These directives should be concise and straightforward. They DO NOT require a lawyer or a huge expense. Many say, "Oh, I had my lawyer draw up a document. It's at home." A large, burdensome, expensive, complicated document in a file at home is of little use on the road with you. Your directives can be addressed entirely with a thoughtful discussion with your family and family physician. Once your physician is aware of your advance directive wishes, he or she can write the order for your medical record.

It can often seem complicated to discuss with your family and physicians what kind of resuscitation you would want in a dire situation. Still, you must have thorough discussions with your family and personal physician regarding these matters BEFORE an immediate need arises. I address it with my patients every year at the annual health assessment physical exam visit, beginning at age 60.

Resuscitation may include, but not limited to, cardiopulmonary resuscitation (CPR), oxygen mask, endotracheal intubation (breathing tube insertion), medications, procedures and more. Other issues arise like feeding tubes, intravenous (IV) fluids etc.

In the state of New Jersey, there are three basic types of advance directives. These are offered as an example but be sure to check the laws in your state.

1. Proxy directive - This is in force when a patient elects a representative (i.e., family member or trusted friend) to make healthcare decisions should he or she become unable to make them.

2. Instruction directives - This is also known as a "living will." These are written directives that spell out which treatments a patient is willing to accept and/or refuse. The circumstances in which they are to be enabled may also be defined in this document.

3. Combined directives - This type has features of both previous directives. A proxy is designated to make decisions, and detailed instructions must be followed accordingly.

Any of the above directive types are appropriate and should detail your wishes.

POLST means Physician Orders for Life Sustaining Treatment. If you do not provide any POLST orders, many states require that every life-sustaining and/or prolonging treatment be utilized unless a physician determines it to be futile. An example of this might be an elderly person in a coma, who is so-called "brain dead," and on a ventilator to breathe for him or her. The organ donation and transplant industry may be more aggressive that we know. "Brain death," is indeed, a whole other complicated matter that requires books of its own. Consider the work of my colleague, noted anesthesiologist, Heidi Klessig, MD (https://www.respectforhumanlife.com).

If you don't wish to be an organ, tissue, or body donor, removing your name from state and national registries is not enough. The Uniform Anatomical Gift Act (UAGA) now states that you must have a specific, documented refusal to donate. Otherwise, according to the UAGA, if you come to a hospital incapacitated, and if family is not 'reasonably available', that is to say, able to be contacted by an organ procurement organization without undue effort and willing and capable to act in a timely manner consistent with existing medical criteria necessary for making an anatomical gift, and there is no documented evidence of the decedent's choice not to donate; the administrator of the hospital 'shall make an anatomical gift of the decedent's body or part.'" New Jersey's statute C.26:-85, 9.a.(1)(h) states: "In the absence of actual notice of contrary indication by the decedent, the administrator shall make an anatomical gift of a decedent's body or part." Your documented refusal should be entered into your electronic medical record, stated in your advanced directives, and made known to your family or healthcare surrogates. A signed, dated, and witnessed wallet card stating your refusal to donate may also be carried.

If there is no advance directive, the patient might exist with the help of machines for years, with little to no chance to regain a meaningful life. Dignity and "meaningfulness" of life and death are different for each person. This is why you must communicate your directives to family and physicians so that you receive only the treatment you would wish for in certain situations.

As long as you remain healthy and of sound mind, you can change your advance directives at any time. For instance, if your health situation or prognosis changes, you may reconsider and have new directives instituted. Always make your physicians and close family members aware of your advance directives so that the healthcare team can follow your wishes in an emergency or extended health challenge.

Chapter Seventeen
Contending with Medical Conditions the HINO Way

"The rule of the artery is absolute, universal, and it must not be obstructed."

–Andrew Taylor Still, DO

Heart and Vascular Disease

Physicians, media, and patients used to refer to atherosclerosis as "hardening of the arteries." The popular notion that it is due to aging is not necessarily the case.

Atherosclerosis results in stiffening of the blood vessels. Plaques (soft plugging material) accumulate in the vessels and attach to the vessel walls. For reasons yet to be determined, some people calcify those plaques, that is, to lay calcium rich material to their surface, which hardens them, hard plaque. Unlike a handyman's wall repair with spackle™, the body spackles but does not sand the resultant down to size. This narrows the opening for blood to pass through, reducing or cutting off oxygen to body tissues. The tissues "cry out," causing pain, or worse, may trigger a myocardial infarction (MI/heart attack) or stroke (CVA/brain attack).

Soft plaques can rupture, releasing small plaque pieces up the line to lodge in smaller vessels causing infarctions. They are instances where blood vessels get plugged up completely and tissue on the other end dies (MI or CVA). Soft plaques, though, can be reduced in both size and health compromise with exercise and a vegan diet. See the work of Drs. Dean Ornish and Caldwell Esselstyn.[1]

Hard (calcified) plaques, on the other hand, have a smoother solid surface and don't tend to rupture. But these plaques cannot easily be reversed. Some people calcify their plaques, while others to not. IV chelation therapy may have a role in reducing the mass of calcified plaques, but clinical results are uncertain.[2]

Many diverse factors can predispose a person to atherosclerosis. Smoking (tobacco cigarettes, tobacco cigars, marijuana/cannabis, etc.) can start or worsen the disease. Whether a poison and toxin are legal like tobacco, or illegal in some states like cannabis, they are poisons and toxins just the same. Legality does not imply safety, efficacy, or tolerability. They only state their legality and tax designation, that's all. Toxins in smoke attack the smooth blood vessel walls, making them rough. These rough walls attract platelets (bags of repair chemicals), plaque and blood clots. Carbon monoxide in smoke blocks the red blood cells' ability to carry life-giving oxygen to the body organs. Quitting smoking is a must to prevent atherosclerosis. As always, with any bad habit, it is better never to start, and it is certainly less expensive!

---

[1] Ornish, D. M., Brown, S. E., Scherwitz, L. W., Billings, J. H., Armstrong, W. T., Ports, T. A., McLanahan, S. M., Kirkeeide, R. L., Brand, R. J., & Gould, K. L. (1990). Can lifestyle changes reverse coronary heart disease? The Lancet, 336(8708), 129–133. https://doi.org/10.1016/0140-6736(90)91656-U and Esselstyn, C. B., Jr. (2017). A plant-based diet and coronary artery disease: A mandate for effective therapy. Journal of Geriatric Cardiology, 14(5), 317–320. https://www.ncbi.nlm.nih.gov/pmc/articles/PMC5466936/

[2] Hasan, S., Parikh, M. A., Trivedi, D. B., Frishman, W. H., & Peterson, S. J. (2025). Chelation therapy in coronary artery disease: Fact or fiction? Cardiology in Review. Advance online publication. https://doi.org/10.1097/CRD.0000000000000871

Hypertension (high blood pressure) increases a person's risk of developing atherosclerosis. The reverse is also true: Atherosclerosis can lead to hypertension. Diabetes Mellitus also causes blood vessel disease. Obesity (being overweight) overloads the body and demands more work from the cardiovascular system. This continues until the heart and blood vessels can no longer meet the demand. Reducing your weight to a normal level can lower the risk of atherosclerosis.

With the advent of home blood pressure (BP) monitoring, it appears that BP is lower at home and higher in more stressful settings, such as a physician's office or medical facility. Some refer to this as "White Coat Hypertension." Many times, physicians and others will give patients a pass for having a BP higher than 140/90 when in a medical setting. Not me. A stress test occurs when you put the heart and vascular system under load conditions, such as exercising. Suppose the mere sight of a physician in a white jacket, so-called "white coat syndrome," constitutes a stress test. I tell patients, "If the sight of or sitting in the presence of me in a white jacket is that stressful, then work life, home life, taxes and every other stressful matter must be worse." In that case, you may need lifestyle changes, weight loss, and perhaps psychotherapy or counseling for anxiety-related illness. This is my opinion and experience.

A family history of atherosclerosis in parents or siblings may increase a person's risk. Males tend to have more atherosclerosis than females. Being of male sex is even considered a risk factor. A sedentary lifestyle, or lack of exercise, is a significant risk factor. Engaging in cardiovascular exercise daily can help lower your risk, normalize your weight, and reduce stress. Caffeinated beverages, such as coffee, tea, and colas, increase blood pressure, sleeplessness, anxiety, and tension.

You cannot change your relatives or change your sex, but you can avoid unnecessary risks for atherosclerosis. Prevention and minimizing your risk will help you achieve your best health.

These will help. Antioxidants, found in vegetables, can help reduce the risk of atherosclerosis. Vitamin D3 (cholecalciferol) 125mcg, vitamin E (alpha tocopherol) 400-800 IU daily, and Vitamin C (ascorbic acid) 1000mg twice a day, reduce the formation of atherosclerosis. Garlic and coenzyme Q-10 can also help.

Diabetes: Monitoring your lifestyle

Diabetes consists of a spectrum of insulin secretion and insulin resistance disorders that include impaired fasting glucose, impaired glucose tolerance, gestational diabetes, type 1 diabetes, and type 2 diabetes. These syndromes may be asymptomatic and therefore often go unrecognized. In later stages, they can be generally characterized by elevated blood sugars, fatigue, excessive thirst, and weight gain. If untreated, patients with diabetes may develop serious complications. These include cardiovascular disease and end-organ damage, such as heart attack, stroke, blindness, and kidney failure. Females have a four-fold cardiovascular disease risk while males have a two-fold risk.

If you bring your blood sugar levels down to normal and minimize your cardiovascular risk factors, you can lead a long and healthy life without significant end-organ damage. Normal fasting blood sugar levels may range from 60 to 99. The standard postprandial blood sugar is taken two hours after a meal. The normal level is less than 140. Patients with blood sugar levels of 140 to 200 are considered glucose intolerant. If that blood sugar is greater than or equal to 200, it is suspicious for diabetes. Non-fasting is defined as occurring after meals (postprandial) or at any time (casual).

These numbers are monitored at home with a portable "finger stick" glucometer. Modern glucometers are now wearable. You can attach them to your posterior arm area. The micro size needle inside enables it to consistently sample blood at give constant readings, never before possible. You and your physician should establish a monitoring schedule for both fasting and non-fasting blood glucose levels. Enter these values on a pocket calendar or your portable computer so that you can discuss them with your physician at each visit. Or, write them down in order as they relate to date and meals by preparing a chart.

A healthy lifestyle is essential to managing diabetes and preventing complications. Exercise, a healthy diet, avoidance of toxins, and compliance with your treatment plan are all critical components in the recipe for success.

Your food choices make a significant difference when it comes to managing diabetes. This is due in part to the fact that the body becomes oversensitive to carbohydrates. These are starches and sugars. Simple carbohydrates come in foods such as soft drinks, white bread, potatoes, and pasta. Certain complex carbohydrates, such as plain steel-cut oatmeal, are better tolerated.

For many, protein is obtained from animal sources like eggs, poultry, and meat. It can also be obtained from low-fat plant sources such as soy products like tofu and soy milk. Fat is a source of nutrition and energy; however, saturated fats and cholesterol from animal sources should be limited or avoided. These include bacon, cheese, egg yolks, and shellfish. Better sources of fat and oils are unsaturated fats such as olive oil, fish, and natural peanut butter.

Lastly, fiber is crucial for maintaining the health of the digestive system. Fiber reduces the risk of diverticulosis and can lower cholesterol absorption. Sources of fiber include whole grains, such as oatmeal and whole wheat bread, as well as high-fiber cereals. Unless your physician directs you otherwise, don't forget to drink six to eight glasses of water every day to help your body work at peak efficiency.

Exercise is crucial for minimizing diabetic complications, as well as for managing weight and enhancing overall health. Stretching and flexibility routines will help you prepare for and warm down from your exercise routine. Engaging in at least 30 minutes of cardiovascular exercise every other day can optimize your body's performance on all levels.

Dietary food choices, meal portions, and eating meals on schedule are crucial components of a diabetes treatment lifestyle. Simple carbohydrates (sugars) need to be replaced by complex carbohydrates and fiber. Simple carbohydrates, like sugars, have a high glycemic index. Watermelon and other melons cause a sharp blood sugar spark upward. This means that the food potently and quickly raises blood sugar when you eat it.

Protein and fat, from plant sources, are best in my opinion. Their intake are also essential. Protein is an integral part of a healthy diet, but in excessive quantities, it can decrease kidney function and bone density. Protein intake should be accompanied by increased water intake to help flush out acids produced by its metabolism, or breakdown.

Saturated fat and fried foods should be avoided. Unsaturated fats and oils, such as olive oil, are healthier choices. Remember: extra virgin olive oil is for dressings and sauces, while whole olive oil is for cooking. Whole olive oil has a higher 'smoke-point' and won't burn when cooking at higher temperatures. Adequate water intake is essential to dilute the blood's sugars and cholesterol, to maintain total body hydration, and to help flush the system, keeping the kidneys healthy.

Tobacco smoke should be avoided. Tobacco smoke contains over 7,000 chemicals. 250 chemical products are known to cause disease. Around 80 of these are known carcinogens. These include tar, nicotine, carbon monoxide, formaldehyde, hydrogen cyanide, benzene, toluene, etc. These poisons and toxins can cause cancer and cardiovascular disease by themselves. Teamed up with poorly controlled diabetes, tobacco smoke causes rapid and extensive blood vessel damage.

Alcohol is a source of calories without other nutritive value and toxic to the liver and other organs like the pancreas and stomach. Alcoholic beverages can also interfere with your medicine.

The diagnosis of diabetes is made through a combination of patient history, physical examination, blood testing, and urine testing. Diabetes requires consistent monitoring and a treatment plan from your trusted physician.

After a diagnosis of diabetes is established, patients should receive education on diabetes management. A visit to the nutritionist is essential. Depending on the severity of your diabetes at the time of diagnosis, medicines may be required. Regular eye care by an ophthalmologist and regular foot care by a podiatrist are part of the plan. Home blood sugar monitoring and regular laboratory blood tests will help you and your physician manage diabetes effectively. Further testing for cardiovascular disease and other health concerns may need to be addressed, as diabetes predisposes patients to multiple problems. Fear not, a plan of care and follow-up can prevent many of the *sequellae* (bad outcomes).

A good preventive game plan is based on establishing a healthy lifestyle that includes a balanced diet and regular exercise, and in some cases, medication. Prioritize your goals and continue to monitor and modify your treatment plan in conjunction with your physician. Taking these actions early on will ensure you have the best opportunity for success. "Play The Long Game" (yet another song reference, this time by my friend John Faye).

Labs and Other Tests

At annual history and physical exams, I often perform screening labs, radiology imaging, or other diagnostic tests. Occasionally, patients may request esoteric, expensive, or research-based tests that are not commonly available or readily accessible. Every test, whether screening or diagnostic, has a cost in terms of dollars, time, and suitability. Each aspect must be carefully considered. Some tests are inexpensive, but others are expensive. Some are "covered" by insurance, and some are not. Some may take longer to perform and can only be administered and run in distant places. Some tests are suitable for simple things, and others may be more complex. Some provide concrete answers, while others may only offer suggestions. All these factors can be a mixed bag for each test. This is why it's not practical or possible to run every applicable test as a screening tool or even as a diagnostic tool. Every test, history point, observation, symptoms, examination finding and tool must be taken in context of the whole patient.

Patients often come in with their ideas of diagnosis and the next clinical steps to diagnosis and treatment. Thanks so much to know-it-all relatives and friends, and of course, the vast expanse of the internet, and now AI, artificial intelligence, "we are all doctors now (again, LOL)."

An adult patient had hurt his knee playing basketball over the weekend, with much younger men, I may add (never a good idea). At any rate, he jumped up, landed, and felt something give in his knee. He had to stop playing and iced his knee that evening. The next day, he came in for an appointment and told the story. Now, his knee was minimally swollen, primarily mobile, and non-tender to palpation. I examined his knee in all directions, using half a dozen specialized functional manual tests. I determined that the muscles, ligaments, and joints were intact and capable of bearing weight. With likely conservative management, rest, and then gradual exercise, he would soon be able to return to play (hopefully against men his age).

He said he wanted an MRI, or Magnetic Resonance Imaging scan, to "check it out inside." With the history of injury, patient's history, physical examination of the knee, it was clear that an X-ray or MRI would not be helpful, but would add to the cost, and not likely to improve the outcome. The patient persisted, "I have insurance. Let's get an MRI." The first rule of insurance is don't pay for anything that it doesn't have to. The second rule of insurance is to deny necessary things through precertification and prior authorization at least once, as many will quit and not persist. (But again, I digress.)

I explained to the patient that the likely damage to the knee was minimal. It would heal with rest and gradual exercise, then he could return to play. I recommended physical therapy (PT) evaluation and treatment, and medication if the pain became more severe. He again persisted for an MRI, although it was likely unnecessary. I explained that his insurance wouldn't pay for it till he tried to rest, PT and meds. He became frustrated, demanding the MRI. I told him that his insurance wouldn't pay as he didn't try conservative treatment and had no signs of significant joint damage. But I could get him a $1,200 MRI for just $450 tomorrow if he wanted to pay cash at a private imaging center. He then responded, "Doc, do I need the MRI?"

It is easy to demand the most and best of everything when you believe you are not paying. This is why direct pay care and testing models work well. Patients self-limit their financial risk through their own unique individual value systems. (A third time, I digress.) That'll be another book, or at least, what I've already written about in Medical Economics[3] from 2003 to the present. Work with your physician to decide which tests are practical, reasonable, customary, and individually applicable to you.

The Mother Gland

The pituitary gland is the mother gland of the endocrine system. It connects to the brain stem and sits in the middle of the skull in *sella tursica*, "saddle of the Turk." It is a truly amazing organ. It performs like the mother of the house. It constantly samples the blood for hormones and other substances, signaling back with its approval or disapproval —a feedback loop.

Here's a typical example. Annually, I frequently screen patients for TSH, or thyroid-stimulating hormone, to test whether a patient may be experiencing chronic fatigue or other related complaints. If the TSH is low, the thyroid gland is likely cranking

---

[3] Medical Economics. (n.d.). Medical Economics – Physician business, practice management coverage. Retrieved August 13, 2025, from https://www.medicaleconomics.com/

out high amounts of active thyroid hormone. This indicates that the thyroid is overactive, (hyperthyroidism). If it is high, then the pituitary is like the mother yelling at the thyroid to make more hormone (hypothyroidism). This is like the mother who signals the kids to do more of the work she has assigned. Who is better at monitoring and directing all the work that goes on at home than Mom? In this way, the pituitary and its hormones and other signals are in charge, and we can benefit by interpreting its actions.

Osteoporosis

Osteoporosis is a progressive condition characterized by the gradual thinning and weakening of bones. Over time, this can increase your risk of significant bone fractures, including the hip and pelvis.

Bone density reaches its maximum by age 35. After that, the body metabolizes calcium from the bone for metabolic processes. As it thins, it becomes osteopenic. This is the first stage of thinning. Osteoporosis is the final stage of thinning, which puts an individual at risk for significant and painful bone fractures. We all know individuals in their elder years who have suffered spine and hip fractures. These bone breakages are consistently painful and often lead to other fractures. The destabilization of the bony structures also predisposes a person to organ disease and dysfunction. Often, the person who developed a hip or spine fracture finds their health going downhill fast due to immobility, pain, depression, and loss of function.

On average, osteoporosis affects more women than men, especially those with a slender, thin-framed build. Osteoporosis is also more common in those whose elder family members had a history of multiple bone fractures or osteoporosis. These bone weaknesses typically result from genetic factors, aging, a lack of weight-bearing exercise, inadequate calcium intake, inadequate vitamin D, and other nutrient deficiencies that can occur throughout a lifetime.

As always, prevention is the best medicine. A healthy diet rich in calcium, vitamin D3, and magnesium is essential for maintaining your bone mass (sturdiness). Supplements can augment a healthy diet rich in low-fat dairy products. Consider taking chelated calcium 600mg once or twice a day, vitamin D-3 (cholecalciferol) 2,000-5,000 IU (125mcg) once daily, and magnesium 1,000mg once daily. Soy products, such as tofu and soy milk, can also be beneficial. They may have a mild estrogenic effect, similar to female hormones, and may help preserve bone.

The National Osteoporosis Foundation (NOF) has specific guidelines to identify those at risk for osteoporosis. Postmenopausal women who have had any type of bone fracture should be tested.

The most well-established bone mineral density test is dual-energy x-ray absorptiometry (DEXA scan). Women over the age of 70 who suffer a fracture can be presumed to have osteoporosis. Testing for these women helps to establish a baseline. This can be used to determine the effectiveness of the treatment over time. The NOF recommends testing for all women aged 65 years and older. I usually recommend a screeing baseline study at 50 years old for women and susceptible men.

Younger postmenopausal women should also be tested if they have one of the following risk factors:

1. Having a parent or sibling who has suffered an osteoporotic fracture

2. Being a smoker

3. Having a low body weight, less than 127 lbs.

4. Being estrogen deficient (e.g., reaching menopause before age 45 or having premenopausal amenorrhea for longer than one year)

5. Having had lifelong low calcium intake

6. Chronic use of steroid medicine (e.g., for asthma or other inflammatory condition)

Early detection of bone thinning is key. A DEXA scan is used to measure bone density. It is a simple and painless test that quickly determines the level of bone density. Once you know this number and designation, you and your physician can treat the problem if necessary. Medicines are available to increase your bone density. In doing so, they can lessen your risk of fracture.

Daily weight-bearing exercise, such as walking, will also help to prevent osteoporosis. Quitting smoking and reducing your intake of caffeinated beverages, such as coffee, tea, and colas, further reduces your risk of this disease. Remember, a healthy lifestyle is key to maximizing your bone strength.

Arthritis

Joint pain and stiffness can be the result of arthritis. There are two fundamental types of arthritis, osteoarthritis, and rheumatoid arthritis. Although both may produce similar symptoms, they differ in their causes and treatments.

Osteoarthritis is a "wear and tear" disease of the joints. As we age, our joint tissues become less flexible. The cartilage cushions in our joints can wear out. Less fluid cushioning is in the joints as we age. All these factors contribute to osteoarthritis. The changes can occur in any joint, including the knees, hips, back, and neck.

In my opinion, much osteoarthritis is caused by excessive weight, poor posture, and other lifestyle factors, which are not only correctable, but preventable. A unique factor that I have determined through more than three decades of Osteopathic family medical practice, and over 55 years of life, is the development of fascial restrictions and scarring over time.

Rheumatoid arthritis is an autoimmune disease. This refers to the fact that, in some individuals, the immune system antibodies will attack joint tissue. This can make the surfaces less smooth and even ragged. In some severe cases, it can cause irreversible damage to the joints, rendering them unusable. Psoriatic and other forms of autoimmune arthritis can be similarly devastating over time.

To differentiate between these and other arthritic conditions, physicians begin with a detailed history. Specific answers to health history and current condition questions can give physicians clues to the diagnosis. Physical exam findings also may suggest a diagnosis. Blood tests and imaging studies (x-ray, CT, MRI) may be used to confirm the diagnosis.

Certain supplements can improve arthritic conditions. Glucosamine and chondroitin are constituents of healthy joints and are available in capsule form. Antioxidants, such as vitamin C and vitamin E, are also helpful in preventing further tissue damage.

Exercise is a critical factor in preventing and even treating various forms of arthritis. Daily stretching and flexibility programs keep the muscles and joints more flexible. Cardiovascular exercise can increase healthy fluid flow to and from joints and other tissues. Prevention and proper treatment will help toward worry-free body performance.

Cold / Upper Respiratory Infection

In modern usage, a "cold" typically refers to an upper respiratory infection. A virus, such as rhinovirus or adenovirus, is primarily responsible for this. It is a virus that affects the nose, throat, ears, sinuses, and upper airways. Symptoms may include sore throat, ear pain, ear popping, sneezing, itchy eyes, runny nose, headache, and cough. A significant fever over 100.5°F is usually not present, hence the name "cold."

The illness is usually self-limited or simply runs its course in two to seven days. It doesn't require antibiotics because they are not effective against the viruses that cause colds. It is a good idea, though, to drink plenty of water and get plenty of rest to help your body's immune system win the battle quickly.

Although no currently known medicine can cure the common cold, people use various remedies to help alleviate the symptoms. Symptom control is essential to most people. They conventionally use over-the-counter cough syrup, decongestants, analgesics, and even antihistamines to reduce the severity of symptoms. Others prefer to use zinc, vitamin C, Vitamin D, and echinacea. Although any of these remedies may or may not help, it is your body's immune system that is responsible for ultimately curing the cold.

Chapter Eighteen
Contending with "Progress"

"New isn't necessarily better."
– Craig M. Wax, DO

Hand Sanitizers?

Since the late 1990s, the personal hygiene industry has marketed "hand sanitizers" and "antibacterial soaps" to the public. I've been sounding the alarm ever since. Although perhaps well-intentioned, hand sanitizers are a plague on our environment. The fact is that weak antibacterial agents, such as triclosan, only kill weak bacteria.

Our world teems with bacteria, which are found on every imaginable surface. What are the most bacteria-laden parts of the body? Would you believe it is your hands? Your hands touch everyone and everything, from handshakes to doorknobs, worsening the concentration and type of bacteria we all carry. We are all protected by most of these harmless commensal bacteria. When they live on our bodies, they protect us from mean bacteria taking their place and causing us risk of disease.

When we use antibacterial soaps and hand sanitizers, we kill off the weak bacteria, allowing ample space and opportunity for pathogenic, disease-causing bacteria to invade. Further, it creates an environmental change if we eliminate those harmless species. We spend our hard-earned money on these products.

From my view, antibacterial soaps and hand sanitizers for routine use are foolhardy. Good old soap and water with a minute of handwashing is the clear winner here.

Technology, Blessing and Curse

The free market has encouraged the development of amazing technological innovations. Is technology a blessing or a curse? Well, yes and no.

With our smartphones, we carry in our hands and wear on our bodies sensors and computers that were unimaginable just a generation ago. We can all have our data connected simultaneously through the internet or the web. Sensors can record, track, and even analyze heart rate, electrocardiac rhythm, blood pressure, blood sugar, sleep cycles, and many other valuable data every day. Is that a good or a bad thing? It is a good thing, in the sense that it provides information and perspective on aspects of your health that you can objectively measure. It is a bad thing if it provides a false sense of security, causes body dysfunction or pain, or the data is stolen or sold without your expressed permission.

Sometimes data about your body is reinforced by "learned" individuals who use podcasts and sophisticated social media to sell you their product or service. The free market gives them space to do this. Your challenge, however, is to discern what is true and useful, and what is meant to frighten you into changing your purchasing habits. If you do not guard against false purveyors of "life-enhancing" ideas, you may not only waste your money, but you will also put your health at risk.

Digital data is already the next generation in communication, employment, management, and government. Digital devices like "smartphones," actually supercomputers, can measure many bits of health-related data.

Fitbit™ started the trend toward reporting health measurement data in the early 2000s by measuring "steps." The company encouraged people to get at least 10,000 steps per day. What does that exactly mean? Not much. Steps were measured by walking with a characteristic arm swing, as the devices were worn as watches. Some people swing their arms more, while others swing them less, during the phases of gait, such as stepping forward and walking—some stroll and some quickly, which makes a difference in calories burned and health benefits. Therefore, "steps" are a rough measure of activity. An active lifestyle with more steps is undoubtedly better than a sedentary lifestyle, but it is no guarantee of health improvements.

Reducing device time and frequency helps minimize pain and dysfunction. Further, daily, and sub-daily neck self-stretches and yoga are self-motivated prevention and treatment schemes. Osteopathic manual medicine (OMM), Chiropractic treatment, and physical therapy can all help when self-treatment does not fix or prevent the problem.

Digital Doctors?

With the digital revolution of the 2000s came the digitalization of your health data at your physician's office. Did patients create this demand? No. Did physicians create this demand? No. Lobbyists, third-party health systems, and the insurance industry convinced the U.S. federal government that the information technology (IT) industry would lead to improved health and care outcomes. The government promised to make ALL your personal private health data available to the entire healthcare ecosystem, but it promised privacy and security.

Congress passed the Health Insurance Portability and Accountability Act (HIPAA) in 1996. HIPPAA took healthcare by storm in the early 2000s. Citizens were told it was "the privacy act" that safeguarded their information in an internet-enabled world. On the contrary, it gave government entities, assignees, and the insurance industry unhampered access to your privileged information, while assigning penalties to physicians and healthcare entities for sharing it as they saw necessary to provide care.

The creation of Electronic Health Records (EHRs) is both a blessing and a curse. On one hand, the professionals who care for you can compile all your health data into one space. On the other hand, in addition to piracy and data loss, the amount of superfluous details can be entirely overwhelming for use in a productive way. The requirement to record everything into each patient's EHR forces physicians to manage digital data entry rather than listening to or examining you! It has turned physicians (MD & DO), nurse practitioners (NP), and physician assistants (PA) into prescribing and refill machines.

Lobbyists and special interests created this "need," which is another example of the tail wagging the boy. They convinced Congress to spend $27 billion to build an EHR system that would allow your personal records to communicate digitally with all the medical professionals who cared for you. Yet, as you read this, government edicts, despite spending billions of tax dollars, have yet to result in EHRs that can seamlessly communicate with each other. This is yet another instance of government by lobbyist cronyism, where the tail wags the dog. We must return to human interaction and unique relationships, to a professional patient-physician relationship.

Since the U.S. federal government intervened in healthcare data transmission, many entities have jumped in to get their share of the healthcare pie. This means that healthcare services now cost you more and pay your chosen physicians less; a losing scenario. It also puts your data at excessive risk for theft, piracy, and outright loss.

The federal government's "gravy train" has led to the emergence of a whole new crop of medical and para-medical facilities. It appears there are urgent care centers on nearly every street corner. Since the passage of the Affordable Care Act of 2010, the number of standalone, urgent care centers has grown 165% to nearly 14,400. [1] One may argue that these provide more and better service to people under medical or mental health stress. Still, they would not exist without the artificial creation of a market driven by tax dollars and imposed government policy. These entities interfere with and disrupt medical care continuity with your trusted physician, all for the sake of convenience.

Smartphone applications (apps) can bring digital healthcare into your hands. If you use them correctly, the data can provide a better understanding of your health at any point in time. However, they miss the mark on the personal human, "analog" relationship with your physician. Are you ready to share your private thoughts and private parts with a random stranger in a new setting, like a clinic or on your smartphone? This is not healthy, and may induce attention deficit disorder, depression, anxiety, or other mental illness. Smartphones and other computerized internet-enabled devices constantly divert our attention from the tasks at hand.

If that weren't enough, now there's Artificial Intelligence (AI). These are computers programmed with algorithms or formulas to sift through millions, and even billions of data points in a few seconds to give you the "best" answer, diagnosis, or treatment. Although it sounds like an advancement, it is riddled with risk. It may be weighted toward more citations of a specific answer, such as democracy, where 51% prevails over 49%, though that 49% may be more correct or wiser. That's why the United States is a representative Republic and not a democracy. But

---

[1] Brilliant Health. (2024, May 12). The marked shift in urgent care utilization: Two years later. Trilliant Health. Retrieved July 18, 2025, from https://www.trilliant-health.com/market-research/studies/the-marked-shift-in-urgent-care-utilization-two-years-later

that's a different discussion and perhaps another book (or see the footnote).[2] AI can be weighted toward certain experts, but this, too, can overwhelm those single sources with potentially the best idea for you. These are just some of the reasons why humans, flawed as we are, are still the single best source for medical consultation, in my opinion.

One solution to this information regulation firestorm is to pursue Direct Physician Care (DPC) a practical and personal form of delivering preventive primary care. In this model, you pay a physician a preset monthly fee for the services that their office provides. It is not insurance but a service contract. Because it is direct, with no middlemen, it is inexpensive. It provides a direct patient-physician relationship where you both understand and know each other. Both patient and physician can count on each other to get through life's troubles, tribulations, and overabundances. This is a natural analog human relationship that may have digital advantages, such as texting and email access.

Bonus: The One Big Beautiful Bill, enacted on July 4, 2025, allows monthly membership fees in a DPC to be tax-deductible if they are paid from a Health Savings Account (HSA).[3] For years, previous administrations had considered these payments to be a form of health insurance ineligible for payment with an HSA.

Technotrauma and iNeck

Since even before 2000, people worldwide have become increasingly enamored of digital devices. Our brain chemistry craves the stimulation (concentration-stimulation theory) of con-

---

[2] Racer, Dave. (2025) *American Government for Real: How We the People Designed our Government to Work.* A&L Publishing, Andover, MN. January 1, 2025.

[3] Section 223(c)(1)(E)(ii)(II): "With respect to any individual for any month, such term [direct primary care service arrangement] shall not include any arrangement if the aggregate fees … exceed $150 (twice such dollar amount in the case of an individual … that covers more than one individual)."

stant interaction. We have adapted ourselves over time to the bipedal, artificial upright position. However, now we have our heads flexed forward, thereby inverting the cervical neck lordosis. This puts all our anatomical structures at a great imbalance and disadvantage. My wife calls it iNeck. I call it technotrauma.

If a healthy life is your priority, you must be mindful of the temptation that comes with iNeck and find better postural ways to interact with this new technology. Are there any inventors out there? Also, too, our eyes are constantly assaulted by artificial "blue light," emitted from these devices. Has the government or anyone done safety studies?

Medical Diagnosis

To better understand the body in disease states, physicians throughout history have described various syndromes in case histories and vignettes. These syndromes sum up disease states where the body or mind is "ill," and cannot function normally to do the activities of daily living, or ADLs. Theoretically, when a person struggles with ADLs, he or she will make an appointment with a physician, healthcare entity, or, if critical, intolerably painful, or potentially life-threatening, with a hospital emergency department. You know my thoughts on that: a person should have an established patient-physician relationship with a private physician for not only urgent or emergent issues, but also routine and opportunistic prevention, to seek and maintain the best health.

As humans, we are constantly under pressure and in a state of flux due to external and internal forces. The external forces are environmental, seasonal, physical, and exposure-based stressors. The internal forces are our defenses, such as our skin, immune system (think of it as an army for fighting external threats and police forces for surveilling and combating internal ones), metabolic processes, and cell turnover, among others. We each have individual, sex-based, familial, ethnic group, cultural, and regional vulnerabilities. Medical professionals use a standard nomenclature, or naming system, to organize and make this disease information useful. It's a disease system, not a health system, FYI.

Using the disease classification system, which is initially based on Latin root words, we name symptom constellations. Examples are Diabetes, Cancer, Arthritis, etc. There are also subdivisions and refinements like insulin-dependent diabetes, prostate cancer, and osteoarthritis. As time passes, further refinements and new names emerge to more specifically describe the syndrome or disease, either by symptoms, behavioral characteristics, or tissue and cell types.

In the 19th Century (1800s), the people witnessed many different movements in health or "medicine:" allopathy, osteopathy, homeopathy, naturopathy, chiropractic, electropathy, hydropathy, and others. With the advent of germ theory, medical professionals shifted their focus toward these microbes as the primary basis of disease. Credit for the discovery and acceptance of germ theory is typically attributed to Louis Pasteur, a French chemist and microbiologist; Joseph Lister, an English surgeon; and Robert Koch, a German physician.

The field of providing health care began to diverge into drug-related forms, like allopathy, and non-drug-related forms, like osteopathy (original doctrine), Chiropractic, Naturopathy, etc. This fracturing led to a schism following the 1910 Flexner report, which was funded by the Rockefeller and Carnegie Foundations.[4] Both organization founders had corporations heavily invested in petroleum, which happened to be the source of the medications, drugs, and treatments they were developing.

---

[4] Flexner, A. (1910). Medical education in the United States and Canada: A report to the Carnegie Foundation for the Advancement of Teaching (Bulletin No. 4). Carnegie Foundation for the Advancement of Teaching.
https://archive.org/details/medicaleducation00flexrich

Abraham Flexner's report purported to standardize medicine and physician practice in the U.S. and Canada. Upon deeper inspection, it served the capital, economic, and industrial goals of Rockefeller and Carnegie, and established the American Medical Association (AMA) as the voice of America's doctors. Flexner's report led to the mainstream adoption of petroleum-based pharmaceuticals. It also served to marginalize all other practices of health and medicine as alternative or fringe.

From the frontier of medical care, Dr. Still predicted that by the end of the 20th Century (1900s), citizens would be inactive, obese, drug addicted (or, at least, dependent), and in poor health.[5] How far was he from that truth?

Here we are, more than a century later, in the 21st century (2000s), with Big Pharma, Big Medicine (encompassing academia, medical schools, and hospital corporations), and Big Government running the "medicine show." The AMA hasn't effectively represented the interests of decent physicians since 1965, particularly in its stance on Medicare and Medicaid legislation. This is where politics began to run, "the medicine show."

Osteopathic medicine (DO) incorporated allopathic (MD) medicine and surgery into its curriculum, while chiropractic, naturopathy, and homeopathy are seen by "the medicine show" as increasingly fringe.

Now, in the present day (2024), people are inactive, morbidly obese (fat), don't eat natural foods, don't drink primarily water, still ingest poisons (caffeine, tobacco, alcohol, cannabis, illicit drugs, don't sleep well, feel depressed or anxious all the time. People take petroleum-based toxins called medications to

---

5 Cody, G. D. W. (2018). The origins of integrative medicine: The first true integrators—the philosophy of early practitioners. Integrative Medicine: A Clinician's Journal, 17(2). https://www.ncbi.nlm.nih.gov/pmc/articles/PMC6396756/ unifacs.br+5pmc.ncbi.nlm.nih.gov+5drkirstie.com+5

accomplish some academic clerical "goal," without addressing their lifestyle shortcomings. Physicians are often incentivized to prescribe medication, rather than spending time helping patients remove barriers to health and improve their lifestyle. This is yet another reason to pay your physician directly, so they work for YOU, not the hospital, medical school, state, federal government, or some other entity with different moral, ethical, and health goals.

It doesn't have to be that way. You don't have to be unhealthy. It is not a fait accompli!

Medications

Medications (drugs), as I mentioned, are selective poisons and toxins, designed to make a profit while potentially making a disease situation "less worse." Certain medications, like insulin for diabetes and thyroid hormone for thyroid disease, have become invaluable staples of the medical arsenal. Although diet, exercise, sleep, and hydration are all critical elements of health, sometimes these dreaded medications are necessary. However, they are generally not a cure, require ongoing monitoring, but may appear to be helpful to produce results beyond essential lifestyle changes, exercise, and weight loss.

There are two basic kinds of medicines, episodic medications, and maintenance medications. Episodic medications can be necessary for a short period, such as antibiotics for 10 days. They can also be "PRN," an abbreviation for "pro re nata," or as circumstances dictate. These can be temporary symptoms, such as reducing medication, like an antihistamine for seasonal allergies, which is taken at the patient's momentary discretion. Maintenance medications are like those used to lower blood pressure, blood sugar, or other long-term treatments.

What if you, under your physician's watchful eye, want to stop a medication? Don't stop any maintenance medication abruptly. Your body is accustomed to having them on board. It's the same for those dependent on the stimulant caffeine in sodas/colas, coffee, tea, and "energy beverages." The body becomes dependent on its daily consumption, and abruptly stopping it will cause a severe headache, often for two to three days.

The way to get off caffeine and, similarly, maintenance medications, is to agree to a plan formulated by your physician and you. The substance must be tapered over days to weeks, depending on circumstances.

Here's a helpful analogy. Imagine checking out a three-story building for purchase as a new home. You walk up the front steps and into the first floor (consider this like taking the lowest dose of a particular medication). You are unsure if there is a benefit here, so your physician recommends going up to the second floor, or middle dosage strength. You haven't noticed side effects but still don't see any benefits. With your physician's guidance, you elevate to the third floor, or the highest dosage strength for this medication. Now, at the top, you either don't notice benefits, experience side effects, or just want to leave. Now, what would you do? Would you jump out of a third-floor window just to leave immediately? Hopefully, cooler heads will prevail, and you will descend, step by step, with your physician's guidance and support. This would prevent falls and potential injuries. Once safely on the first floor, you could go down the front steps to the yard and decide on your next move. (You are now free from the harmful effects of the stimulant that has been causing you trouble, or the ineffective medication.)

The pharmaceutical industry and entire supply chain create and market new chemical compounds with a goal in mind and a target audience. They then invest a billion dollars and ten years, generally, to pass Food and Drug Administration (FDA) rules for "safety and efficacy." There are two divergent problems:

1. Big pharma heavily invests in FDA regulators and members of Congress to make the rules fit the research and company interests, not just the research to fit the rules as initially intended. "Drugmakers spent a record $31 million to lobby in Washington last year, and about $13 million in the first quarter of 2025." [6]

2. FDA government administration, rules, and regulations are so bloated that a product can be slowed to a stop and even eliminated, while the pharmaceutical company hemorrhages money, time, and resources. It is a regulatory mess, sometimes called "regulatory capture."

Drugs and genetic interventions get unjustly passed through the regulatory gamut while good medications are economically killed in the dragged-out process. Science is bought and sold to the highest bidder or those with the most significant political influence. The Centers for Disease Control (CDC) is no better for similar reasons. Many government agencies are compromised in this way.

Take, for example, branded and generic medications. Branded medications, in their first year of FDA-approved product life, must recoup all research and development costs accrued over 7 years as the company "built" the new drug. This results in a high price and an expensive product. Generic medications cost pennies to produce but cannot be marketed until the pharmaceutical company's patent expires. In the first year of generics, prices do not drop significantly because the FDA limits the market entry of generics for one to two years after the brand's patent expires. This causes prices to remain high.

---

[6] Dawsey, J., Peterson, K., & Severns, M. (2025, April 30). Drugmakers have spent millions targeting 'middlemen'—and it's paying off. *The Wall Street Journal.*

After that, many generic medications, varying in quality, strength, and potency, may come on the market. Those generics, however, can vary by 20% or more in amount and potency compared to the branded counterparts. That represents a total variance of 40% from the original. This is why many physicians demand the brand name for insulin and thyroid medications. Then the insurance company, along with its henchmen, the Pharmaceutical Benefit Managers (PBMs), gets involved to deny payment for the brand because a cheaper generic is available. It is even more heinous, as the PBMs restrict access to the formulary, which the insurer owns.

Who gave insurance companies and PBMs this power? It was the federal government, as you've probably guessed. They allow PBMs to extort the pharma manufacturers for kickbacks, which they call "rebates." The federal government extended a "safe harbor" from the anti-kickback statute to PBMs in 2003, during the George W Bush administration. The original safe harbor was for General Purchasing Organizations (GPOs) in the late 1980s.

These returned monies, called "rebates," are supposed to be returned to the insurance plan sponsor, employer, or patient, but they do not. They are maintained by the PBMs, who have compelled companies to include their formulary on the drug menu for plan sponsors, employers, and patients.

It would be great if we all rose up in protest and took the fight to our elected state and federal officials to repeal the GPO safe harbor and its extension to the PBMs in 2003, thereby reintroducing competition instead of corporate Marxism, which is what we have now. (Yes, this has a lot to do with you achieving and maintaining a healthy life.)

Attitude

"The union of the natural forces that constitute the body of man is vastly superior to the capacity of any artificial force."
–Andrew Taylor Still, DO

A positive attitude goes a long way to achieving and maintaining your optimal state of health. Media frequently tell stories of people who "beat the odds," cured cancer or some other malady with the power of positive thinking. Although there are many helpful therapies and treatments available, they are magnified tenfold when the power of a positive attitude is part of the regimen.

The mind-body connection was discussed in the chapter on Stress. The attuned mind can detect most stressors and minimize responses to them. This conserves energy and leaves you better prepared to face life's daily challenges with a smile.

By merely using simple visualization techniques, a person can transform their whole world. Imagining yourself in a more suitable place, job, relationship, or state of health can be the most effective first step toward achieving it. Of course, a reasonable step-by-step plan is the next key factor.

Changing the way you think about things and tasks can change the outcome from your actions. For instance, I hated shoveling snow as an adult. As a kid, I could make a few bucks shoveling out neighbors. But, as an adult, husband, father, physician, and business owner, snow looked like a pending expense, and it threatened the safety of our staff, patients, and family. My wife feels insecure walking on snow, ice, and slush due to a previous slip and fall. Now, what should I do? My mind said to ignore it and wait until it melted in the spring.

One day, I decided to reconsider snow as an opportunity to get another hour of biceps and back exercise by shoveling at dawn. Now, I prepare the night before and equip myself with a personal music player, warm, dry clothes, waterproof boots, and strong, warm mittens. On snow days, I get an extra hour of exercise for personal health and get to help my family out of a jam; it's a win-win.

Motivation is one of the keys to unlocking our optimal health. We need to maintain a strong positive motivation to change our lives. We also need to feel happy with what we have. That is best explained by the "smelling the flowers" principle. "You got to stop and smell the roses / You've got to count your many blessings every day…"[7]

Every day, we all need to express happiness with the things that we value in our lives: loving relationships, faith, music, flowers, art, pride in our work, a sense of achievement, respect for others and their beliefs (even if they differ from our own).

[7] Mac Davis, Doc Severinsen. (1974). Stop and Smell the Roses." Columbia Records and the composers.

Chapter Nineteen
Poised for Success

"Ipsa scientia potestas est" ("Knowledge itself is power")
— Sir Francis Bacon, *Meditationes Sacrae* (1597)

Sir Francis Bacon wrote that knowledge is power. It is especially true if you use that knowledge, especially self-knowledge, to your ultimate advantage.

Always set yourself up for success whenever possible. Know your strengths, limitations, and weaknesses.

Whether you're religious, agnostic, atheist, or anything in between, there is a famous Bible verse from Matthew 6:13 that is a valuable principle for everyone: "And lead us not into temptation, but deliver us from evil." This is undoubtedly useful for consideration. Even the ancients knew how difficult it was to fight human inclination.

The ancient peoples recognized that humans are drawn to certain things by powerful forces, whether in the universe or within our own bodies. We know that neurochemistry, along with its genetic and environmental programming, can significantly affect our day-to-day activities, bodies, and lives. Why do you think that the supermarket puts candy, gum, and magazines in the checkout lanes? They are so-called impulse buys that may be hard to resist. We didn't come into the store for them, but they piqued our biochemical interest along the way. And, in the checkout lane, there's not much time to reconsider and put it back down.

Don't set yourself up for failure! The phrase "If you can't take the heat, get out of the kitchen" is often attributed to former U.S. President Harry S. Truman. Don't put yourself in a position to fail. If you can't resist ice cream, don't go to the ice cream shop and don't walk through the frozen dessert section of the supermarket.

Patients often hear me say, "I have enough willpower to say no, thank you, but I don't have enough willpower to say no more, thank you." Many of us can't be led to temptation, or worse, just have a taste of something, actual or metaphorical. This can lead to the beginning of a slippery slope to failure, accompanied by negative emotions, bad feelings, and destructive thoughts. Here it comes again, the backbiting monster of REGRET!

If you can't resist gambling, don't go to the casino for dinner. I would no sooner go to a casino for dinner and a show if I could not walk passed gambling machines and table games. The same goes for alcoholic drinks in a bar with live music; the object of my affection. Point of clarification; live music is the object of my affection, certainly not alcohol caloric toxin.

"If you can't say no, don't go!" – Craig M. Wax, DO

Take Control and Responsibility

"Whether you think you can, or think you can't – you're right."
–Henry Ford

Getting healthy and staying healthy is that simple. Be enthusiastic! You will see results in just a few days, and the positive consequences will be lifelong. Apply the simple ideas presented in this book to your lifestyle and start winning the constant battles of id, ego, and superego. Individuals can live meaningful lives and overcome many challenges. So, why not you? Get started right now!

How many psychologists does it take to change a light bulb? Only one, but the light bulb must want to change! That old joke is axiomatic and dogmatic. Primarily, you can only change yourself. Take stock and get started. You can do this.

"Jim" is a 75-year-old patient who always comes into the office with a smile and a positive attitude. He came in one day with gauze bandage wrapped all around one of his hands. It made his hand look like a white boxing glove. In the exam room, I inquired as to what it was and what had happened. Jim said that he was working in a machine shop, and his third finger was immediately amputated, and his hand was now sewn up and bandaged (quite noticeably!). He was still smiling through the retelling of events, and I thought this peculiar. I asked Jim why he didn't seem angry, sad, or even upset about the traumatic loss of his finger. He said, "Dr. Wax, I could have lost my whole hand!" Wow, what a positive perspective! Are there injuries and personal losses in your life that you might reframe and reconsider?

"John" is an 82-year-old friend and patient of mine (living a good life in his elderhood). He embodies most, if not all, of these principles. He is vital, full of life, and all who meet him believe he is 20 years younger than he is. John walks three to five miles a day, has a low-fat, low-processed-sugar, high-fiber diet, and drinks plenty of water. He is undoubtedly making the best of his genetics and his environment.

John's good health practices helped him get through a tragic accident. One day, a tractor-trailer truck broadsided John's car, with him in it. John sustained a subdural (brain) bleed and many broken ribs. With time (three months) and a gentle return to his good habits, he resumed living his normal state of health. Joe is truly a fantastic individual. We all have similar health and recovery capabilities if we all subscribe to the basic principles of maintaining health.

Like anything else that you want to accomplish, you must make health a priority, or disease will find you. As magical as modern medicine may seem, the best medicine is prevention. Choose not to be ill. Choose health. Health is number one!

Dr Wax's ten rules for human wellness:

1. Drink water, not "drinks."
2. Eat food, not "junk."
3. Go to sleep early and rise early.
4. Exercise daily for at least one hour; don't be lazy.
5. Practice relaxation and meditation daily.
6. Don't poison yourself.
7. Treat people the way that you want to be treated.
8. Apologize when necessary.
9. Read and learn new skills.
10. Set health goals and achieve them.

Observation, experience, lessons learned, and opinion

"He who reigns within himself and rules passions, desires and fears is more than a king."

— John Milton

As a family physician for over three decades, through being observant and listening to patients, I've learned many valuable lessons.

The first lesson learned is that patients seldom do what you tell them to do unless they are interested, motivated, and have some ownership in the patient-physician relationship, having bought into the process. Like parenting our offspring, patients don't do what you tell them but may do what you show them by what you do in your own life. For example, I follow a vegetable-based diet, drink primarily water, get adequate sleep at night, and exercise for an hour or so a day at sunrise. I share my current activity with patients, so they know that good healthy habits are possible, despite daily home and work responsibilities.

Another lesson learned is not to tolerate the excuse, "WE ARE ALL BUSY!" As a husband, father, and a physician who practices family medicine, a school physician for two districts, a published author, an award-winning media host, a board member of a physician organization, a follower of breaking medical trends and medications, and many other interests, I make time for my health first. That's where it all begins and ends.

Another thing that I've learned as a physician and father is that children are resilient; so are patients. Even teenagers, growing, emotional, boundary-negotiating, and making mistakes(!) are incredibly resilient. Often, pediatricians and family physicians must treat the parents more than their children. Always start by speaking to the children with respect, giving them your full attention, maintaining eye contact, and using a calm tone. Treating them as individual people who matter is crucial not only to their success but also to your success as a parent or caregiver.

This book represents a compendium of my observations, experiences, lessons learned, and opinions. I wish you well on your life's health journey. Determine your meaning, find your path, pursue your dreams, and achieve success and happiness. But first, and foremost, be well!

"Understand your own nature first and you'll begin to harness your own power."

– Craig M. Wax, DO

Contact Craig M. Wax, DO

Dr. Wax's website:

https://HealthIsNumberOne.com

Social Media: @drcraigwax

Instagram
Facebook
X
LinkedIn
Truth Social

Correspondence:

Craig M. Wax, DO
155 North Main Street
Mullica Hill, New Jersey 08062

Made in the USA
Coppell, TX
22 June 2026

83152258R00105